KNOW THE FACTS

THE FACTS ABOUT
Vaccines

Andrea C. Nakaya

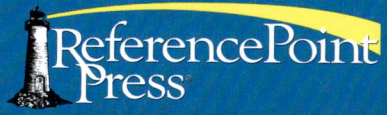

San Diego, CA

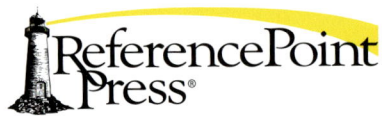

© 2026 ReferencePoint Press, Inc.
Printed in the United States

For more information, contact:
ReferencePoint Press, Inc.
PO Box 27779
San Diego, CA 92198
www.ReferencePointPress.com

ALL RIGHTS RESERVED.
No part of this work covered by the copyright hereon may be reproduced or used in any form or by any means—graphic, electronic, or mechanical, including photocopying, recording, taping, web distribution, or information storage retrieval systems—without the written permission of the publisher.

LIBRARY OF CONGRESS CATALOGING-IN-PUBLICATION DATA

Author: Andrea C. Nakaya
Title: The Facts About Vaccines
Description: San Diego, CA : ReferencePoint Press, 2026. | Series:
 Know the Facts
 Includes bibliographical references and index
Identifiers: LCCN 2025005195 (print) | ISBN
 9781678210441 library binding | ISBN 9781678210458 ebook

For compete cataloging-in-publication data please go to www.loc.gov.

CONTENTS

Introduction 4
A Public Health Triumph

Chapter One 8
How Important Is Vaccination?

Chapter Two 20
Vaccine Side Effects

Chapter Three 31
Vaccine Safety

Chapter Four 42
Vaccine Mandates

Source Notes 54
Organizations and Websites 57
For Further Research 59
Index 60
Picture Credits 64
About the Author 64

INTRODUCTION

A Public Health Triumph

In December 2019, the coronavirus disease 2019 (COVID-19) appeared in China and spread rapidly from country to country. This virus proved lethal to many people; in the United States alone, a million people died during the first two years of the COVID-19 pandemic. In addition, hospitals struggled to care for the hundreds of thousands of patients who needed urgent medical care. The virus was so frightening that many people were afraid to leave their homes for fear of catching it, and governments were quick to order citizens to refrain from going out to work, shop, or gather. Life dramatically changed for nearly everyone on the planet. A few months into the pandemic, high school senior Noelle Johnson commented, "This is one of the hardest things that my generation has had to deal with."[1] Then, in late 2020, scientists announced that they had developed a vaccine for COVID-19. That vaccine was distributed around the world and immediately altered the course of the pandemic. According to a 2024 study published in the *Lancet* medical journal, COVID-19 vaccines have saved millions of lives. The researchers report that between December 2020 and March 2023, the vaccine reduced US deaths by 59 percent, which equals 1.6 million saved lives.

> "This is one of the hardest things that my generation has had to deal with."[1]
>
> —Noelle Johnson, high school senior

Vaccines are widely considered to be one of the greatest accomplishments in the history of public health. The COVID-19 story is just one example of how they can help save millions of lives and dramatically reduce the spread and effects of severe illness. However, despite the success of vaccines, these medicines have always provoked debate too, and hesitancy and outright opposition have grown in countries around the world in recent years. Vaccines have become the subject of controversy, and many people have strong opinions about them. For those trying to make sense of the controversy, it can be helpful to separate the facts from the many emotions present in the debate.

How Vaccines Work

Vaccines function in connection with the immune system. The body's immune system is constantly working to protect a person from bacteria, viruses, and other germs that can invade and multiply, causing sickness. When the immune system detects an invading germ, it releases antibodies to fight that germ. This response might take some time, and a person may end up getting sick in the process; however, after the germ has been destroyed, the immune system will remember both the germ and how to make the antibodies that will destroy it. If the same germ ever tries to attack again, the immune system is ready and can quickly release the necessary antibodies, destroying the germ and protecting the person from getting sick. This is known as immunity.

Most vaccines cause immunity by imitating an infection. They contain a very small amount of dead or weakened germs, which initiate an immune response. This response might cause a person to feel slightly unwell for a day or two but does not make the body suffer the symptoms of a full-blown infection. It might take several weeks—or, in some cases, multiple doses of the vaccine—but a person eventually develops immunity to the germ they have been vaccinated against. In recent years, scientists have also developed a new vaccine technology—called messenger ribonucleic acid (mRNA)—that helps a person develop immunity by giving their cells instructions for making antibodies rather than injecting dead or weakened germs.

The first vaccine was developed in 1796 by English physician Edward Jenner. It was for smallpox and immediately provoked both praise and skepticism. At that time, smallpox was deadly, killing approximately one in three people who caught it. Patients developed fluid-filled lesions, or "pox," over their entire bodies, and those who survived were often left disfigured or even blind from the lesions. Many people were thus eager to be vaccinated against this disease. However, at that time, much less was known about germs and disease, and there was also a lot of fear and skepticism of Jenner's vaccine. For instance, some people were afraid of putting a foreign substance into their bodies, others believed it was unchristian, and some even believed that vaccination was useless because, in their mistaken view, smallpox was caused by "bad air" or supernatural forces. Eventually, the vac-

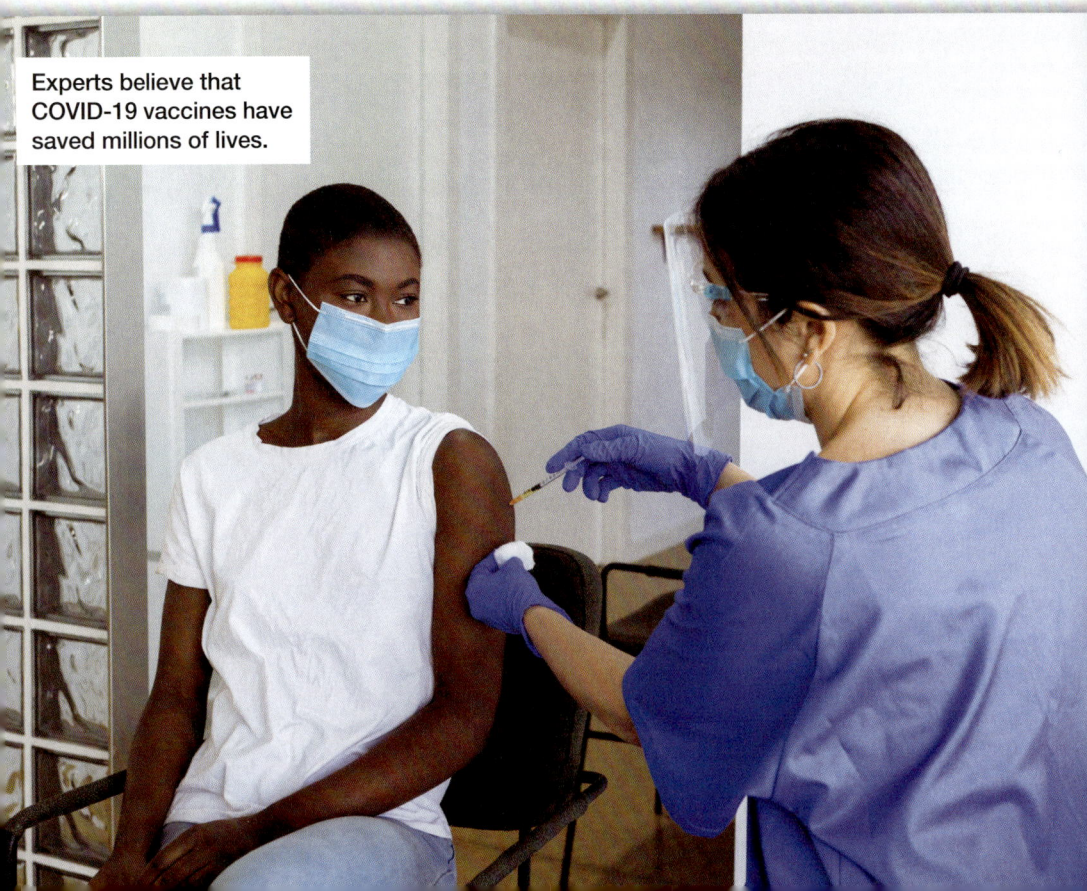

Experts believe that COVID-19 vaccines have saved millions of lives.

cine was proved to be safe and effective, and its success was copied around the world. Jenner's discovery led to the eradication of smallpox—a monumental medical achievement.

Ongoing Controversy

Over the years, numerous vaccines have been developed and used on people, but with each one, there is debate over safety, efficacy, and ethics. Some concerns are based on facts. For instance, there are many peer-reviewed research studies that reveal the potential side effects of specific vaccines and how common these effects are. Medical organizations such as the Centers for Disease Control and Prevention (CDC) also provide factual vaccine-related information. However, many vaccine-related debates are not based on fact. For instance, some people are opposed to vaccines based on stories that they have read on social media or heard from friends. There are also many emotional stories on both sides of this debate. These are commonly based on personal experience but not backed by scientific evidence. In addition, there are many outspoken advocates and critics influencing the vaccine debate, including celebrities and politicians, who can be extremely persuasive but are not medical experts. Sometimes their voices are amplified over the medical community and repeated on social media platforms by fans. All these competing opinions can make it challenging to separate facts from speculation. However, taking the time to read vetted news sources and understand how vaccines and other medicines function can reassure people that vaccines do work and have prevented illnesses from spreading unchecked and claiming numerous lives.

CHAPTER ONE

How Important Is Vaccination?

Polio is an infectious disease caused by a virus. It affects the nervous system and can lead to paralysis of the arms, legs, or muscles used for breathing—and can even be fatal. Polio most often strikes children. During the late nineteenth to early twentieth centuries, polio outbreaks were common in the United States and many other countries, particularly during the summer. Large numbers of children who became infected were paralyzed and ended up needing crutches, braces, or wheelchairs for the rest of their lives. Some even had to use an iron lung, which was an artificial respirator that helped them breathe.

At that time, nobody knew what caused polio. Parents were terrified that their children would catch it. They checked them constantly for symptoms, often kept them away from crowded public places like swimming pools or sporting events, and told them not to play with children they did not know. Cathy, who contracted polio when she was two and a half, became one of the thousands of US children who were paralyzed by the disease. She had to have numerous surgeries on her foot, wear leg braces that made it difficult to walk, and go through months of therapy. She says,

> I always had limitations. I couldn't ever do what everybody else did. I couldn't wear certain shoes because they just didn't fit right. I couldn't keep up with other kids. I've never been on roller skates since my one foot does not go

straight; it just turns outward. Playing jump rope was an issue, but I tried my best because I was stubborn. And I pushed forward and pushed myself, and I was able to ride a bike, but some of it was tough trying to keep up.[2]

During the 1950s, US physician Jonas Salk created a successful vaccine for this terrible disease. The vaccine was licensed in 1955, and widespread vaccination began immediately. By 1994, polio was eliminated from North and South America, and families no longer had to live in fear of their children dying or becoming paralyzed from the disease.

The Benefits of Vaccination

Many vaccines have significant benefits. As the history of polio shows, vaccines help reduce the number of people who suffer from the long list of serious health complications that can be caused by certain preventable diseases. Polio is just one example of a disease that can be prevented by vaccination. Others include meningococcal disease, which can result in deafness or developmental disabilities; hepatitis B, which can cause liver disease; and rubella, which can result in brain infections or lead to miscarriages or birth defects in pregnant women. Karen Sadler was born partially deaf after her mother contracted rubella during pregnancy, and she eventually became completely deaf. She says,

> "I always had limitations. I couldn't ever do what everybody else did."[2]
>
> —Cathy, polio survivor

I was born with some hearing in my left ear. My right ear never ever heard. Over time, I lost the little bit of hearing that I had. . . . When I finally got my hearing aid in the summer between seventh and eighth grades, I turned to my mom and said, what's that sound? And she started crying because that was the first time I had actually heard a bird. There were lots of things I didn't hear. I couldn't hear wind or anything with high frequency. And if you know, female teachers in schools are all high-frequency voices. That made it difficult to hear and understand in many of my classes.[3]

Many of these diseases can also cause death, which means that by preventing infection, vaccination has also saved the lives of millions of people. The World Health Organization (WHO) estimates that over the past fifty years, vaccination has saved 154 million lives globally, which is equal to 6 lives every minute. "Vaccines are among the most powerful inventions in history, making once-feared diseases preventable," says Tedros Adhanom Ghebreyesus, director general of WHO. "Thanks to vaccines, smallpox has been eradicated, polio is on the brink, and with the more recent development of vaccines against diseases like malaria and cervical cancer, we are pushing back the frontiers of disease. With continued

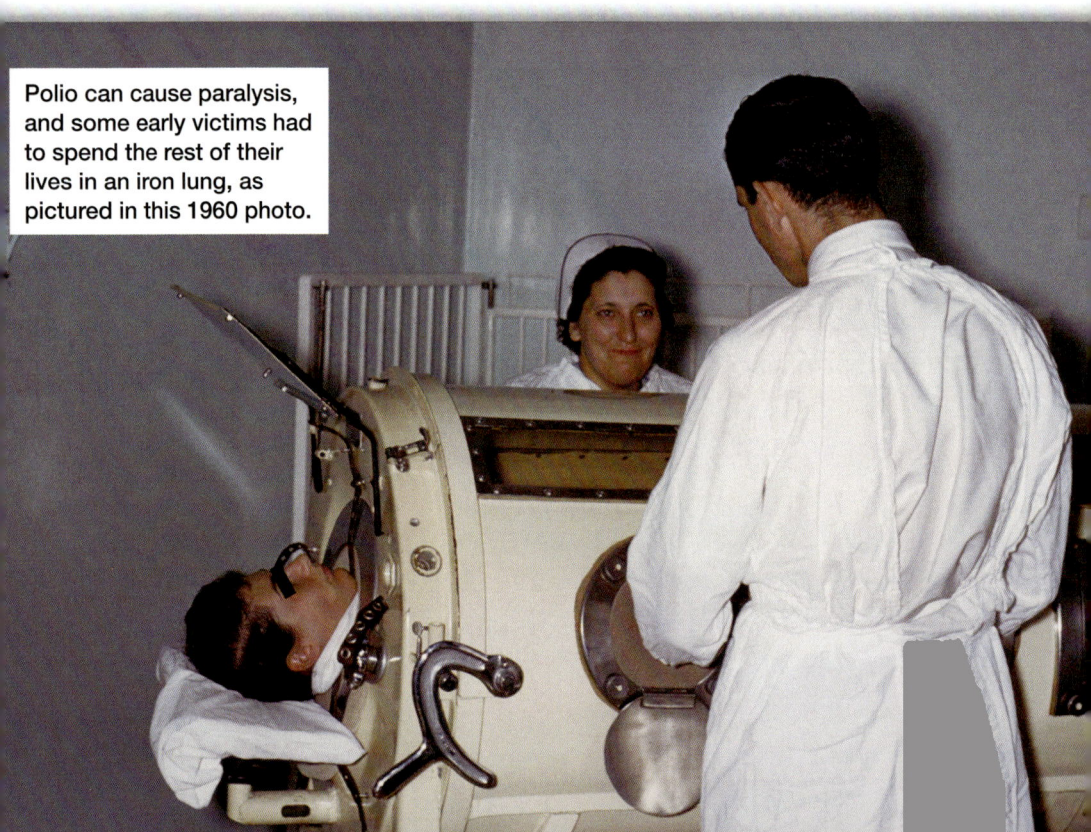

Polio can cause paralysis, and some early victims had to spend the rest of their lives in an iron lung, as pictured in this 1960 photo.

research, investment and collaboration, we can save millions more lives today and in the next 50 years."[4] Many of these lives belong to infants. WHO reports that infant deaths have been reduced by 40 percent globally because of vaccination. Catherine Russell, executive director of the United Nations Children's Fund, comments, "Thanks to vaccinations, more children now survive and thrive past their fifth birthday than at any other point in history."[5]

> "Vaccines are among the most powerful inventions in history, making once-feared diseases preventable."[4]
>
> —Tedros Adhanom Ghebreyesus, WHO director general

Vaccination also has economic benefits. Because it reduces the number of people who get sick, it helps lessen medical expenses, including the cost of doctors, medicine, and hospital care. It also reduces the economic losses that result from sick people being unable to work. The National Foundation for Infectious Diseases (NFID) explains that many diseases are very costly. According to the NFID, "Diseases have a direct impact on individuals and families, and also carry a high price tag for society as a whole, exceeding $10 billion per year."[6] For instance, the NFID says that on average, a person who gets the flu can be sick for two weeks and is likely to miss at least a week of school or work. It reports that hepatitis A is associated with a whole month of missed work.

Community Benefits

When people get vaccinated, there are also benefits for their communities. After many people in a community are vaccinated and become immune to a particular disease, that disease is much less likely to spread, meaning that the risk of illness is lessened for everyone. This is often referred to as herd immunity. Herd immunity protects weaker members of a community who are more vulnerable to getting sick. This includes young children, the elderly, and people who have weak immune systems, such as cancer patients who are undergoing chemotherapy. Herd immunity also benefits people who cannot be vaccinated. For example, people who have certain serious allergies may not be able to receive certain vaccines. Those with weakened immune systems, such as people with human immunodeficiency virus (HIV) or acquired immunodeficiency syndrome (AIDS), are another group who may not be able to get vaccinated. Herd immunity can also protect infants who are too young to be fully vaccinated. WHO insists that everyone who can be vaccinated has a responsibility to do so for the sake of the community. It says, "We would think it irresponsible of a driver to ignore all traffic regulations on the presumption that other drivers will watch out for them. In the same way, we shouldn't rely on people around us to stop the spread of disease; we must all do what we can."[7]

Ultimately, consistent community vaccination can lead to the eradication of a disease. The only disease that has been completely eradicated this way is smallpox. However, there are many other diseases that are now very rare in certain places because

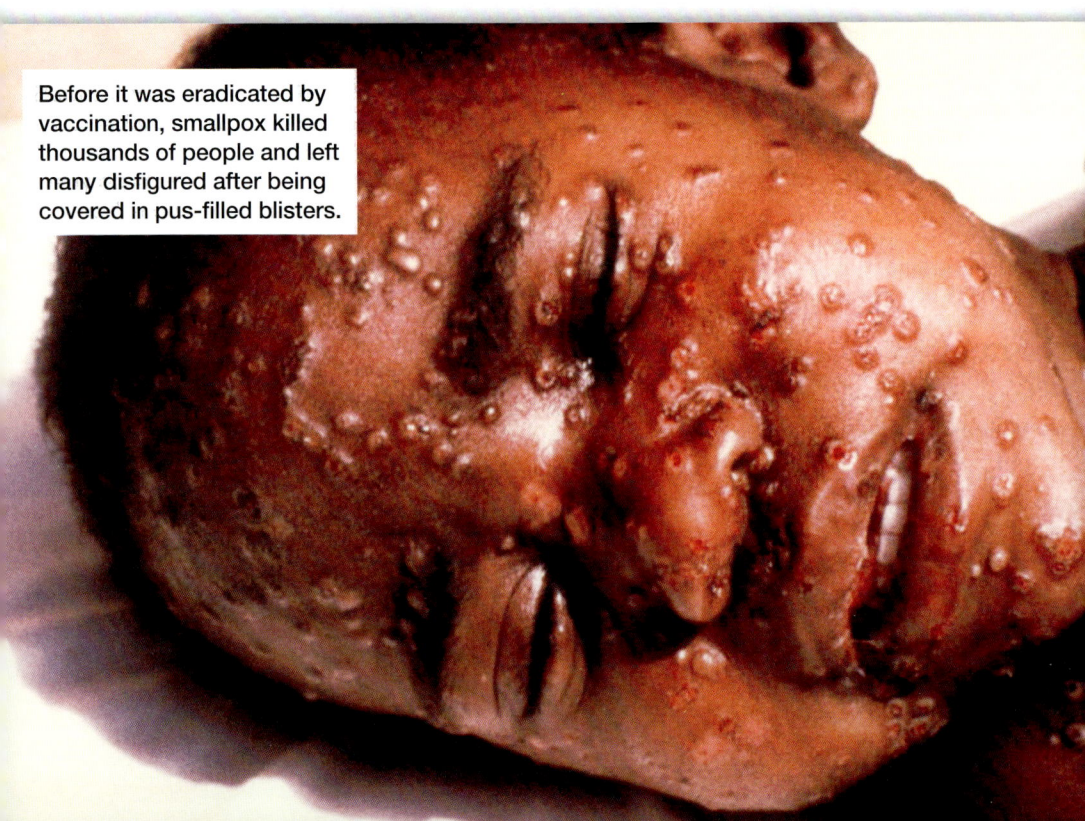

Before it was eradicated by vaccination, smallpox killed thousands of people and left many disfigured after being covered in pus-filled blisters.

large numbers of people have been vaccinated against them—meaning they cannot spread easily within communities. Diphtheria is one disease that used to be common but has become rare in many parts of the world. This disease can result in heart failure, paralysis, and death. According to the CDC, diphtheria sickened hundreds of thousands of people in the United States during the 1920s and 1930s. Vaccination for diphtheria began in the 1940s, and the CDC reports that the last reported US case was in 1997.

Relying on Herd Immunity

Some people choose not to vaccinate themselves or their children because of the existence of herd immunity. They rely on the fact that most of the people around them have been vaccinated and are thus immune to a particular disease, which means that disease is unlikely to be present in the community. The problem with this approach is that if too many people rely on herd immunity, it will disappear. For instance, public health experts estimate that to achieve herd immunity to measles, 95 percent of the population needs to be vaccinated against this disease. They say that if less than 95 percent vaccination is achieved, the virus will be able to find enough unvaccinated people to infect that it can survive within a community.

Another problem with relying on herd immunity is that it cannot be achieved with some diseases. COVID-19 and the flu are examples of this. Because they continually mutate, lasting immunity is difficult to achieve. This contrasts with the measles virus, which does not change much over time. With measles, herd immunity is possible because people only need to catch the disease once or get one series of vaccinations and they have lasting immunity.

Is Vaccination Always Best?

There are a lot of benefits associated with vaccination; however, there are also a lot of questions regarding how important this form of protection is. For instance, many people wonder whether it is better to catch a disease and develop natural immunity rather than becoming immune by receiving a vaccine. There is no doubt that in most cases, natural immunity does provide strong protection against illness. Numerous studies have been conducted to determine which type of immunity is best—natural or vaccine-derived—but researchers have been unable to discover a definitive answer. There is evidence that for some diseases, natural immunity lasts longer. For example, most people who are infected with mumps become immune for life. In contrast, mumps vaccination does not seem to result in lifelong immunity. The CDC says that for people who receive the measles, mumps, and rubella (MMR) vaccine, immunity can decrease over time, and they might still catch mumps later in life. It explains that "some vaccinated people may still get measles, mumps, or rubella if they are exposed to the viruses. It could be that their immune system didn't respond as well as they should have to the vaccine; their immune system's ability to fight the infection decreased over time; or they have prolonged, close contact with someone who has a virus."[8] However, even if natural immunity does last longer in some cases, experts point out that it can be riskier to acquire because it involves actually becoming sick with a particular illness. For example, the mumps virus is relatively mild for some people, but it can cause serious complications in others, including loss of hearing and infertility.

Another common question about vaccination is whether it is still necessary for people to continue to get vaccinated against certain diseases in places where these diseases have been eradicated or have become rare. Critics argue that in such cases, the risk of contracting these diseases is much lower than the risks associated with potential side effects of taking the vaccine, so it may be better to skip the vaccine. Vaccine advocates contend that unless a disease has been eradicated worldwide, there is always

Does Having Had COVID-19 Eliminate the Need for Vaccination?

It is true that people who get sick from COVID-19 and then recover will have some immunity to this illness. However, scientists are not sure exactly how strong a person's immunity is after infection or how long it lasts. In addition, the virus that causes COVID-19 continues to change, which means that infection from one variant might not result in immunity to a different variant. The Cleveland Clinic reports that there is also evidence that the strength of immunity varies depending on the variant that infected a person. It says that newer variants may not provide immunity that is as strong or long-lasting as earlier variants, explaining that "these newer variants have 'high immune escape.' This means they're sneaky and can more easily dodge your body's natural immune defenses." As a result of all these factors, most experts recommend vaccination, even if an individual has previously contracted COVID-19. These vaccines are continually being updated to keep up with the virus's mutations.

Cleveland Clinic, "Natural Immunity," August 15, 2024. https://my.clevelandclinic.org.

the chance of a resurgence, which means that vaccination is still a good idea. At present, certain diseases that have been eradicated in some countries are still common in others, and since the world has become increasingly globalized and connected, it is easy for a disease to spread from one country to another. WHO explains, "Travellers can unknowingly bring these diseases into any country, and if the community were not protected by vaccinations, these diseases could quickly spread throughout the population, causing epidemics there."[9]

Why Do Some Vaccinated People Still Get Sick?

Most people who get vaccinated are protected from getting sick, yet vaccination does not always prevent illness. A very small percentage of people get sick even though they have been vaccinated. According to the US Department of Health and Human Services (HHS), there are a few different reasons for this. The HHS says sufferers might have had an underlying medical condition, or their body might have been trying to fight off another serious illness when they got vaccinated. Another possible reason is that the vaccine was not a perfect match for the virus to which they were exposed. This can happen with the flu vaccine. Flu viruses are different every year, and scientists do their best to anticipate which vaccine will be most effective, but they are not always correct. In addition, the effectiveness of certain vaccines wears off over time. An example of this is pertussis, which is commonly called whooping cough. The CDC website has information about the effectiveness of the two whooping cough vaccines used in the United States: DTaP (diphtheria, tetanus, and

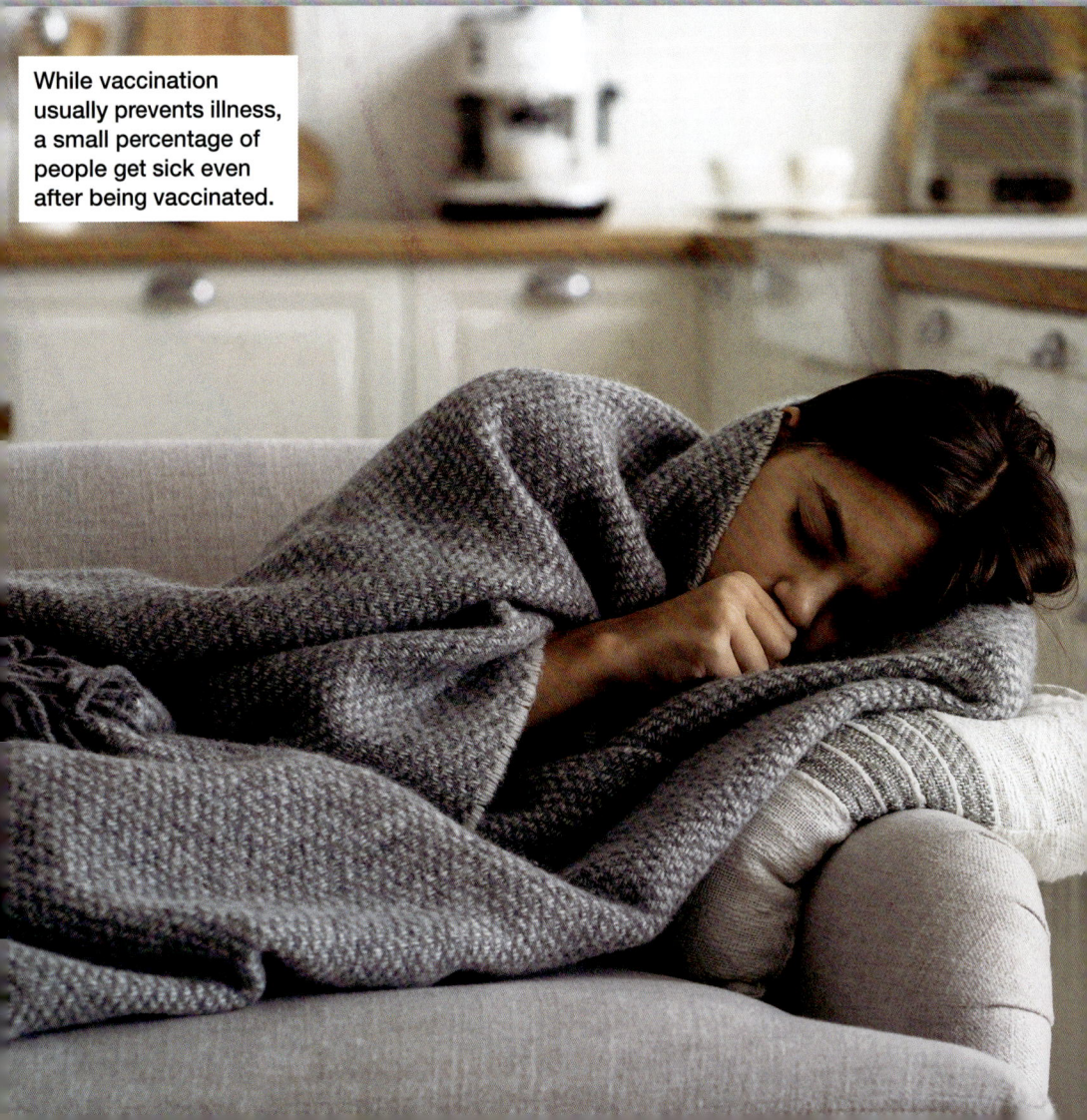

While vaccination usually prevents illness, a small percentage of people get sick even after being vaccinated.

pertussis) and Tdap (tetanus, diphtheria, and pertussis). These statistics reveal that a significant percentage of people who get vaccinated are no longer protected from illness only four or five years after receiving the vaccine. The CDC reports that for children who get all the recommended DTaP vaccinations, almost all are protected for a year after getting their last shot; however, five years later only seven in ten are protected. For Tdap, the CDC states that seven in ten people are protected from illness in the first year, and only about three or four in ten are protected four years after getting the vaccine. However, while not everyone who is vaccinated will avoid becoming sick, vaccination can still be beneficial. The HHS says, "Few things work 100% of the time, including vaccines. Most people will be protected but some may still get sick. . . . But even if a vaccinated person does get sick, the illness is likely to be much less severe than if they had not been vaccinated."[10]

Some people worry that vaccination itself can cause them to catch an illness. This is unlikely, but not impossible. Certain vaccines are made from dead viruses or bacteria, and it is not possible to become sick from these types of vaccines. However, others—such as the MMR vaccine and the chicken pox vaccine—are made with live viruses that have been weakened (also referred to as attenuated). It could be possible to get sick from one of these vaccines, but experts stress that in most cases, the illness would be much less severe than if a person became infected naturally. It is also important to remember that immunity often takes weeks to develop following vaccination, and many vaccines require more than one dose to be effective. As a result, people might believe that they got sick from a vaccination when they simply caught the disease naturally, before their vaccination had time to become effective.

> "Even if a vaccinated person does get sick, the illness is likely to be much less severe than if they had not been vaccinated."[10]
>
> —US Department of Health and Human Services

Access to Vaccination

Whereas some people debate the importance of vaccination, others wish they had the luxury of choice. In some places, people cannot choose vaccination because they simply do not have access to vaccines. According to the United Nations Children's Fund (UNICEF), Africa has the most unvaccinated and undervaccinated children in the world. UNICEF reports that in 2021, 12.7 million children in Africa were undervaccinated, which means they did not receive all recommended childhood vaccines, and 8.7 million of them did not receive any vaccines. The World Health Organization reports that "one in five children in Africa still do not receive all the necessary and basic vaccines. Every year, approximately 30 million African children fall sick from vaccine-preventable diseases, and half a million of them die as a result."

Regional Office for Africa, "Immunization," World Health Organization. www.afro.who.int.

Public Opinion on Vaccination

Attitudes regarding the importance of vaccination have varied significantly over time. In recent years, the percentage of Americans in favor of vaccination has been declining. For instance, Gallup polls show this trend. Gallup conducts regular surveys about attitudes toward vaccination. It reports that in 2024, only 69 percent of Americans said that it was "extremely important" or "very important" for parents to have their children vaccinated, compared to 94 percent in 2021. One possible reason for the decline is that widespread vaccination has caused certain diseases to become rare and they are no longer seen as a serious risk. This means that some people are less likely to see vaccination as important. "When was the last time you heard of someone being hospitalized for measles or a child dying of rubella disease?" asks infectious disease specialist Aniruddha Hazra. He explains that "because vaccines have been so effective at eradicating or really reducing the causes of death for children, people started to question why they were getting a vaccine if they weren't even seeing [the disease]. In that sense, vaccines have been the victims of their own success."[11]

Although certain diseases—such as measles and rubella—have become uncommon in the United States and many other parts of the world, they are no less dangerous. All the vaccines that exist today were developed because the illnesses they protect against represent a significant harm to society. Experts recommend vaccination because they believe it is a vitally important tool for protecting public health.

CHAPTER TWO

Vaccine Side Effects

In 2021, Philadelphia resident Rebeca Cruz-Esteves received her first dose of the COVID-19 vaccine. About four days later, she says that she began to have heart palpitations, followed by muscle spasms, twitching and stiffness in her legs and arms, and a feeling of hyperactivity. Memory fog, excessive thirst, rashes, and reduced eyesight in one eye followed. Cruz-Esteves says that she saw multiple doctors, and none could figure out what was happening to her. "I couldn't sleep," she says. "It was like electricity was running through my body, this jolt . . . and I couldn't feel fatigue, which was very strange."[12] Eventually, doctors diagnosed her with Guillain-Barré syndrome (GBS), which they believe was triggered by her COVID-19 vaccination. GBS is a disorder in which sufferers' immune systems damage their nerve cells. It causes muscle weakness and can also result in paralysis. In most cases, people recover completely; however, some experience long-term nerve damage. GBS is a very rare side effect associated with some vaccines, including the COVID-19 and flu vaccines. Although vaccine side effects like GBS are statistically rare, vaccines do have both risks and benefits, and it is a good idea to fully understand what those are.

Negative Side Effects

Vaccine side effects are rare; however, they do occur in some people. In most cases, negative side effects are very mild and might include pain or swelling at the injection site, tiredness, chills, a mild fever, a headache, or muscle and joint aches. Medical experts say that these side effects are a sign that the vaccine is working and that the body is starting to build immunity against the disease. Yet they add that the vaccine can also work without causing side effects, so people should not worry if they do not experience side effects. Jonathan Jarry, a science communicator for the Office for Science and Society at McGill University in Quebec, talks about one of his vaccination experiences that involved side effects: "Many years ago, I received the flu shot for the very first time and, later that day, I began to feel sick. Fatigue, body temperature on the rise and a general unease made me think I actually had the flu. 'Why get a flu shot if it's going to give you the flu?' I thought at the time." However, Jarry explains, "it turns out that my reaction to the flu shot was natural. It did not give me the flu."[13] Instead, he maintains that his symptoms were likely a result of his body working to build immunity to the flu.

> "Many years ago, I received the flu shot for the very first time and, later that day, I began to feel sick."[13]
>
> —Jonathan Jarry, a science communicator at McGill University in Quebec

More serious side effects are statistically rare for most vaccines. However, in a very small percentage of people, vaccines can cause a severe allergic reaction, serious health problems, or even death. Allergic reactions occur in individuals who are allergic to something in the vaccine and can range from minor to life-threatening. According to the HHS, out of a million people who receive a vaccine, one or two might have a severe allergic reaction. Symptoms of an allergic reaction include having trouble breathing, a rapid heartbeat, swelling of the face and throat, a rash, and feeling dizzy or weak. Other types of serious reactions to vaccines vary depending on the vaccine. For instance, according to the CDC, only 1 or 2 in every 100,000 people in the United States will get GBS. Most of those cases are not even the result of vaccination but are caused by something else, like an infection, surgery, or serious trauma. Another example of a serious vaccine

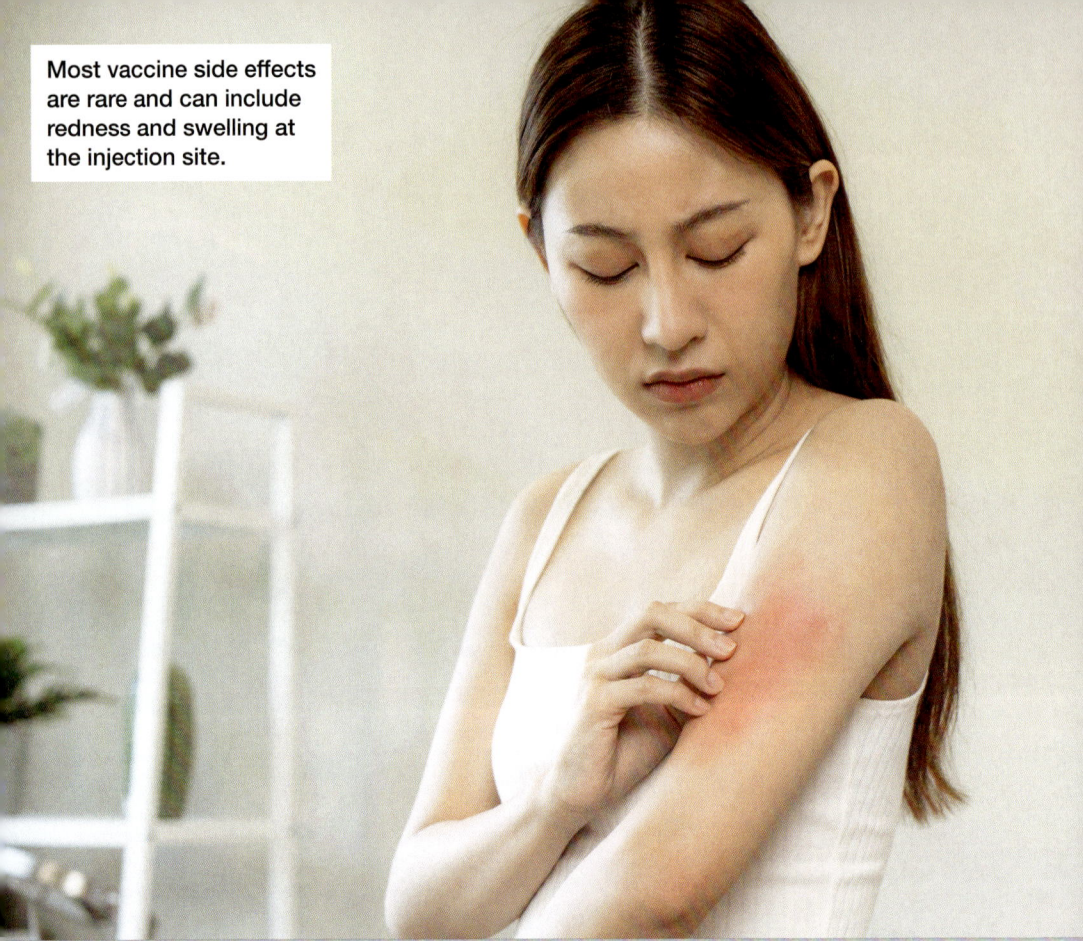

Most vaccine side effects are rare and can include redness and swelling at the injection site.

side effect is encephalitis, which is swelling of the brain. Overall, according to WHO, "more serious adverse events occur rarely (on the order of one per thousands to one per millions of doses), and some are so rare that risk cannot be accurately assessed."[14]

The fact that these side effects are rare, however, makes them no less harmful to the people who do experience them. Tina, a mother from Portland, Oregon, tells a story of the serious nature of vaccine side effects. She reports that her eighteen-month-old daughter experienced several health problems after receiving three different vaccinations against a total of six different diseases. She says that her daughter began by having trouble walking, then progressed to vomiting up her food

> "More serious adverse events occur rarely (on the order of one per thousands to one per millions of doses)."[14]
>
> —World Health Organization

at every meal. Soon after that, she had a seizure. Tina shares the experience, for which her own mother was also present. She says that her mother called 911, and the paramedics took her daughter to the emergency room. She explains,

> In the ER she had her blood drawn and was clearly upset, screaming. While they were trying to catheterize her (to get a urine sample) she started screaming again and proceeded to have another seizure. She was taken to have a CT [computed tomography] scan and then admitted to the hospital. . . . She was weighed and re-dressed and while on mom's shoulder, she was crying and not settling down. It was then that she had another seizure.

Her daughter did eventually recover, but Tina says that when she looks back at the official report she submitted regarding her daughter's reaction, "I weep over seeing this and feel every second unfold like it was yesterday."[15]

Estimating exactly how many people experience side effects from vaccines can be difficult because in many cases it is impossible to know whether a health problem was caused by a vaccine or simply happened at the same time as the vaccination. One way to get a better understanding is to look at reports of adverse events that people believe are related to vaccines. Tina reported her daughter's side effects through the Vaccine Adverse Event Reporting System (VAERS), which is a government website where people can report adverse vaccine reactions. According to VAERS data, in 2024, about 49,000 total adverse events were reported in the United States. However, it stresses that these have not been verified; anyone can report an event, even without proof that it was caused by vaccination. Another way to learn how common vaccine side effects are is to look at statistics from the Vaccine Injury Compensation

Program, a government program through which people can file a petition for compensation from a vaccine-related injury. Only certain vaccines are covered under this program. (Claims related to the COVID-19 vaccine are covered under a different program). The Health Resources and Services Administration (HRSA) reports that between 2006 and 2022, 5 billion doses of covered vaccines were distributed. It says that there were 12,499 adverse event claims resolved by the court, with 9,075 compensated. According to the agency, "This means for every 1 million doses of vaccine that were distributed, approximately 1 individual was compensated."[16]

COVID-19 Vaccine Side Effects

There have also been reports of side effects associated with the COVID-19 vaccine. *New York Times* journalist Apoorva Mandavilli spent a year investigating COVID-19 vaccine side effects. Her research included interviewing people who said they had suffered from serious side effects. She recounts some of their stories. For instance, she says, "Renee France, 49, a physical therapist in Seattle, developed Bell's palsy—a form of facial paralysis, usually temporary—and a dramatic rash that neatly bisected her face." In another example, "Dr. Ilka Warshawsky, a 58-year-old pathologist, said she lost all hearing in her right ear after a Covid booster shot."[17] Janet Woodcock, the principal deputy commissioner at the US Food and Drug Administration (FDA) between 2022 and 2024, said in an interview that while adverse reactions to the COVID-19 vaccine are rare, they have been "serious" and "life-changing" for some people. She added, "I feel bad for those people."[18]

People who believe they have been harmed by the COVID-19 vaccine can file a claim through the Countermeasures Injury Compensation Program. According to data provided by the HRSA, as of December 1, 2024, more than thirteen thousand claims had been filed for compensation for harm from a COVID-19 vaccine.

Is It Dangerous to Give Children Multiple Vaccines at Once?

Most of the vaccines that people will receive over their lifetimes are administered when they are young. In the first few years of their lives, children visit the doctor frequently, often receiving four or five different vaccines in one visit. By the time they are two years old, a child might have received more than twenty vaccines. Some people worry that this is too much and could overwhelm a young immune system. Experts contend that the suggested immunization schedule for children is based on extensive research and has proved to be the best way to protect children from all these diseases. In response to worries about overwhelming the immune system, they point out that young children are constantly doing things that expose their immune systems to different antigens, or germs. In a blog article for the Spokane Regional Health District, the author explains,

> As soon as babies are born, their immune systems start going to school. They begin learning how to recognize and eliminate tiny invaders—like viruses and bacteria. . . . And let's be real, babies are *constantly* exposed to new things. Anything they put in their mouth (which is basically anything that they can grab), or even just the dust they breathe, is like a mini lesson in "How to Identify Antigens 101." They're basically walking classrooms for germs.

Amy Jennings, "Do Babies Get Too Many Vaccines?," Spokane Regional Health District, December 12, 2024. https://srhd.org.

So far, there have only been decisions on a small number of those claims, with only sixty-two people being found eligible for compensation.

While the possible side effects associated with the COVID-19 vaccine and other vaccines can be frightening, contracting many of these diseases can result in lingering illnesses. For example, some people who catch COVID-19 later suffer from something known as long COVID, which can last for months or even years. This is a chronic condition that has a long list of possible symptoms, including fatigue, brain fog, shortness of breath, trouble sleeping, and chest pains. For some people, these symptoms are so long-lasting and severe that they are unable to continue with work or school. Eric Bossward tells his long COVID story:

> The fatigue had become just unbelievable. I couldn't think properly. I was suffering from horrendous breathlessness, as well as dizzy spells. I also had the most horrific anxiety, waking up every morning with an overwhelming sense of dread. . . .
>
> At my worst, I felt suicidal because of it. Nobody wants that. If you can do anything to protect yourself from getting COVID-19 in the first place and so avoid the risk of it developing into long COVID, then my message would be to definitely do it.[19]

Although estimates vary, some studies show that at least 5 percent of US adults have suffered from long COVID. Vaccination is believed to reduce the risk of long COVID. Addition-

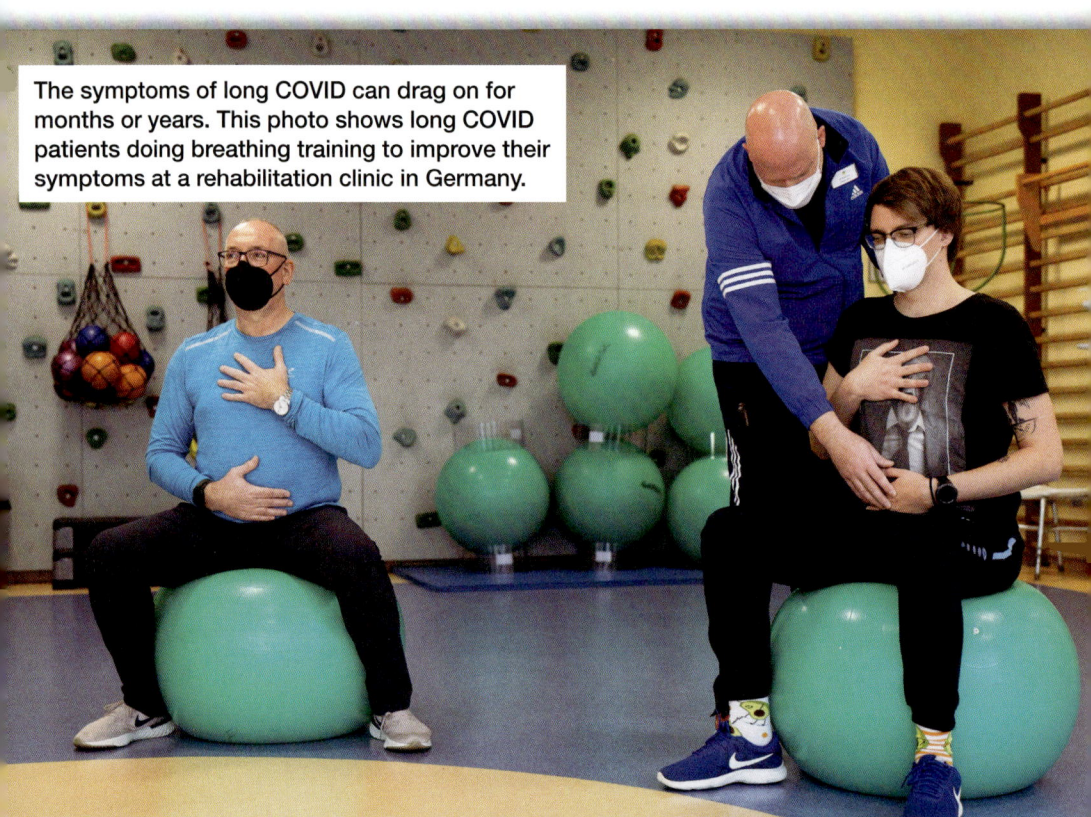

The symptoms of long COVID can drag on for months or years. This photo shows long COVID patients doing breathing training to improve their symptoms at a rehabilitation clinic in Germany.

ally, while some people choose not to get vaccinated because they do not want to risk the potential side effects, certain illnesses can cause the same health problems anyway. For example, some studies have shown that people with the COVID-19 infection many develop GBS.

> "If you can do anything to protect yourself from getting COVID-19 in the first place and so avoid the risk of it developing into long COVID, then my message would be to definitely do it."[19]
>
> —Eric Bossward, long COVID patient

The Safety of Vaccine Ingredients

When it comes to vaccine side effects, some people worry less about the active vaccine ingredients but more about the other ingredients that are added to vaccines. For example, some vaccines contain preservatives to stop the growth of bacteria or fungi. Some include what are known as adjuvants, which are substances that are added to help a person have a better immune response. Others contain ingredients that are used to inactivate viruses so that they will not give a person the disease that they are being vaccinated against. Some of the ingredients added to vaccines do have the potential to be harmful in large doses. For instance, formaldehyde is an ingredient commonly used for inactivating viruses, and research has shown that exposure to large amounts of this chemical may cause cancer. Some vaccines also contain thimerosal, which is used as a preservative. Thimerosal contains mercury, which has also been shown to be harmful to health at high levels.

However, experts stress that these ingredients are important to the safety of vaccines; for instance, they prevent vaccines from going bad. In addition, experts stress that just because something is harmful at a high dose does not mean it is harmful at the very small dose present in a vaccine. For instance, the FDA points out that people already have formaldehyde in their bodies because the human body continuously produces this chemical. It explains,

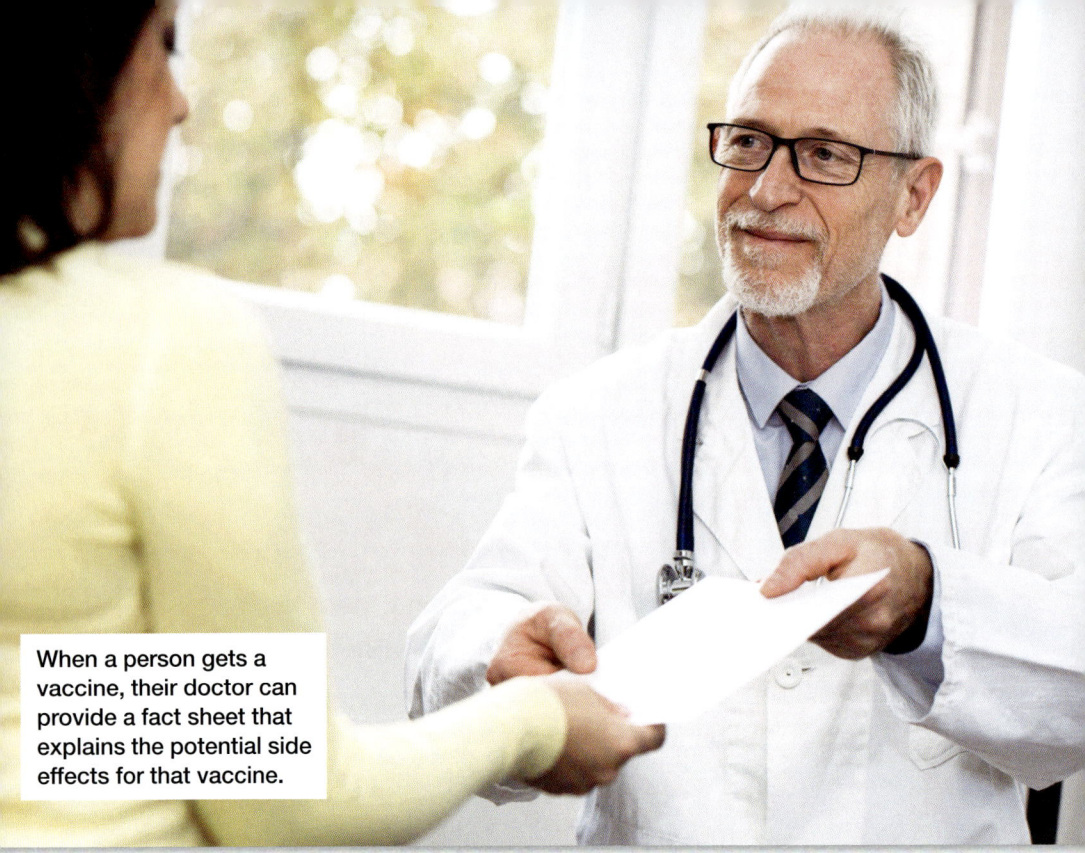

When a person gets a vaccine, their doctor can provide a fact sheet that explains the potential side effects for that vaccine.

"Studies have shown that for a newborn of average weight of 6-8 pounds, the amount of formaldehyde in their body is 50–70 times higher than the upper amount that they could receive from a single dose of a vaccine or from vaccines administered over time."[20] The American Academy of Allergy, Asthma & Immunology similarly highlights thimerosal. It explains that thimerosal is also present in vaccines in tiny amounts that are lower than what people are naturally exposed to from other sources and is unlikely to pose a health risk. It stresses, "Any substance can be harmful in significantly high doses, even water."[21]

The MMR Vaccine and Autism

In some cases, people worry about vaccine side effects that lack credible evidence of occurring in recipients. One of the best examples of this is the MMR vaccine. In 1998, British physician and researcher Andrew Wakefield and his colleagues published a study in the *Lancet*, a well-respected medical journal, arguing that there was a connection between the MMR vaccine and autism. The study quickly ignited panic around the world and caused many parents to opt against giving their children the MMR vaccine because they did not want them to develop autism. Researchers later found that the study was invalid. They discovered that the children Wakefield had studied had not actually developed autism because of the MMR vaccine but had simply developed it at around the same time as they were vaccinated. The study was retracted from the *Lancet* in 2010, and authorities revoked Wakefield's medical license. In addition, several studies have been conducted since then that have shown no link between the MMR vaccine and autism.

However, even though it was proved false, Wakefield's s study has had a lasting impact on attitudes toward vaccination. Before the study results were discredited, they were publicized around the world, fueling widespread skepticism of the MMR vaccine. Many

The COVID-19 Vaccine and Heart Issues

While side effects from COVID-19 vaccines are relatively rare, some people—particularly young people—have experienced myocarditis after getting an mRNA vaccine (the Moderna or Pfizer vaccines). Myocarditis is inflammation of the heart muscle. According to the Centers for Disease Control and Prevention, this side effect is most common in adolescent and young males and usually happens within a week of their second mRNA COVID-19 vaccine. In most cases, myocarditis can be treated with medication and rest; however, in a small number of people, it has caused long-lasting symptoms, such as chest pain and shortness of breath, which have prevented them from doing many of their normal activities. As a result, some young people have been afraid to be vaccinated. Experts maintain that vaccination is still safer because COVID-19 infection can cause myocarditis too, and it is usually more severe and longer lasting than what results from vaccination. Professor of immunobiology Akiko Iwasaki explains, "With infection, you not only get myocarditis, but you also get all these other symptoms and damage to your lungs and other organs. You could also develop long COVID."

Quoted in Isabella Backman, "Q&A: What Causes Rare Instances of Myocarditis After mRNA COVID-19 Vaccines?," Yale School of Medicine, May 16, 2023. https://medicine.yale.edu.

parents refused the vaccine for their children. For years afterward, even when the study had been retracted, a lot of people continued to refuse the MMR vaccine. Even today, many remain suspicious of it because of the publicity surrounding Wakefield's study.

Risks Versus Benefits

When vaccines are tested, researchers report on all observed side effects. Even after a vaccine has been approved, monitoring of side effects continues. The CDC publishes a fact sheet for every vaccine that it recommends, which lists potential side effects. These fact sheets are available online and from most medical providers. In addition to side effects, the fact sheets list reasons for getting that vaccine, the recommended vaccination schedule, when a person might want to talk to their health care provider before getting a vaccine, what to do if there is an adverse reaction, and where to look for more information about vaccination.

Vaccine side effects can be scary, but they are only part of the story. Experts argue that in deciding whether to receive a vaccination, every individual needs to weigh the potential risks against the potential benefits. WHO stresses, "Looking at risk alone is not enough; you must always look at both risks and benefits." Most medical experts believe that for the majority of people, the benefits of vaccination outweigh the risks. They argue that although all vaccinations come with a small risk of side effects, vaccination is significantly less risky than catching a particular illness. Most of the diseases that vaccines protect against can also cause substantial harm. Like most public health agencies around the world, WHO concludes, "While any serious injury or death caused by vaccines is too many, it is also clear that the benefits of vaccination greatly outweigh the slight risk, and that many, many more injuries and deaths would occur without vaccinations. In fact, to have a medical intervention as effective as vaccination in preventing disease and not use it would be unconscionable."[22]

CHAPTER THREE

Vaccine Safety

The average vaccine takes ten years or more to develop. Researchers and manufacturers must follow a long list of steps that are designed to ensure safety. In contrast, the first approved COVID-19 vaccine was developed in a record-breaking eight months. When the vaccine was approved, millions of people around the world lined up to receive it. However, there was also widespread skepticism. One group of researchers surveyed people about their perceptions of the vaccine. They found that many worried it might not be safe because of the fact that it was developed so quickly. For instance, one person said, "I'm no scientist but I always believed vaccines took years to make and get right and develop and test."[23] Another commented, "I think it was done too fast, and I think as a result the preparation wasn't done."[24]

Experts stress that all of the standard safety procedures were followed in developing the COVID-19 vaccine. They explain that the speed of development was possible due to a combination of advances in vaccine technology and the cooperation of scientists, manufacturers, approval boards, and regulatory agencies. In addition, tens of thousands of people were anxious to volunteer to participate in clinical trials, which also helped accelerate development. Yet despite the many strict rules governing the development of the COVID-19 vaccines and others, vaccine safety is something that a lot of people worry about.

The First Vaccine

The first successful vaccination was carried out in 1796 by English physician Edward Jenner. Jenner vaccinated eight-year-old

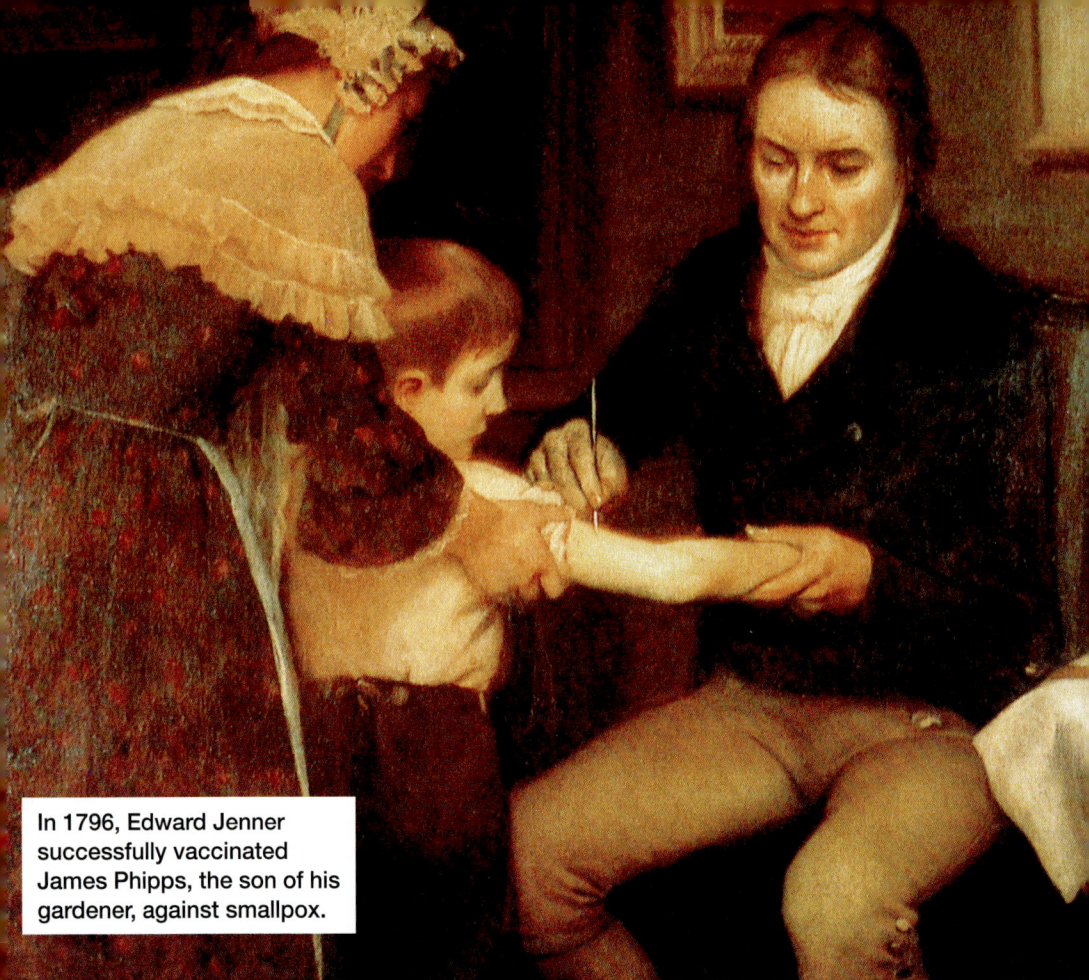

In 1796, Edward Jenner successfully vaccinated James Phipps, the son of his gardener, against smallpox.

James Phipps, who was the son of his gardener, against smallpox. Jenner did this by making scratches on the boy's arm and then rubbing the cowpox virus into the scratches. Cowpox is a similar virus to smallpox, and Jenner had noticed that people who had suffered from cowpox did not catch smallpox. His theory was that vaccination with cowpox would be similar to naturally catching this illness and would give Phipps immunity to smallpox. Phipps became mildly ill but quickly recovered. Jenner then deliberately infected the boy with smallpox to see whether the vaccination had worked. His experiment was successful, and Phipps did not get sick. However, Jenner had conducted a potentially fatal experiment on a child, which is something that is considered highly unethical today. He went on to experiment on more children, including his infant son. Once he determined that his technique was effective, he attempted to vaccinate as many people as possible. According to a British Broadcasting Corporation article, "He converted a rustic summerhouse in his garden into his Temple of Vaccinia and invited local people to be vaccinated after church on Sunday."[25] He also encouraged other physicians to do the same.

The Process of Developing a Vaccine

The process of testing, producing, and administering vaccines has become far more strictly regulated than it was in Jenner's time. In the United States, vaccines are regulated by the Center for Biologics Evaluation and Research, which is part of the FDA. The CDC explains that for most vaccines, there are seven steps for development: research and discovery, proof of concept, testing, approval, the manufacturing process, recommending the vaccine for use, and monitoring safety after approval. The first step, the research and discovery phase, takes place in a laboratory and can last ten to fifteen years. In this first phase, researchers try to gain a better understanding of how a particular infectious organism makes people sick and then they work to develop a vaccine for it. Not all vaccine research is successful. For example, despite trying for many years, researchers have still been unable to develop a vaccine for HIV.

The next step in the process is called proof of concept. In this phase, researchers test their potential vaccine on mice or other small animals to see whether it causes an immune response. At this point, they can adjust the vaccine to make it safer and more effective. If animal trials show that the vaccine works, researchers move on to clinical trials, where the vaccine is tested on people. Testing is generally done in three phases, though in some cases, there is a fourth phase. In the first phase, the vaccine is given to small groups of less than one hundred people, and researchers study its effects and monitor any side effects. Phase two expands testing to groups of one hundred to three hundred people, with researchers gathering more information about how well the vaccine works and any side effects that occur. In phase three, testing is expanded to groups of one thousand to three thousand people. Phase four, if it occurs, takes place after vaccine approval, and thousands of people are studied over a longer period so that researchers can get an even better idea of the effectiveness and safety of the vaccine. While phase three trials are being conducted, the FDA also evaluates the proposed vaccine manufacturing process and facility to ensure that the company producing it will be able to reliably and consistently manufacture large amounts of the vaccine. In addition, it tests several batches of the vaccine to make sure that each one is the same.

Finally, the vaccine manufacturer can apply for approval from the FDA. It must submit information about testing and manufacturing, which is then reviewed by the agency. The FDA may also look at input from the Vaccines and Related Biological Products Advisory Committee, which is an independent scientific committee that will review data about the safety and effectiveness of the vaccine. If the FDA approves the vaccine, large-scale manufacturing can begin. An additional step is recommending the vaccine for use. To do this, health experts consider many different factors, including the safety and effectiveness of the vaccine and the seriousness of the disease that it prevents.

After approval and recommendation, there is continual oversight of vaccine quality and of the manufacturing facility. In addition, the FDA continues to monitor the safety of the vaccine, including through the VAERS website, where people can report adverse reactions. Every country has its own process for developing and monitoring vaccines; however, most follow a similar process that includes extensive testing and continual monitoring.

Safety Failures

Despite all the rules and processes designed to ensure vaccine safety, there have been times when the process has failed. The

A COVID-19 Hero

Katalin Karikó is a Hungarian American biochemist whose research was a critical part of the successful development of the COVID-19 mRNA vaccine. She spent much of her career researching mRNA technology, and without her work, the quick development of a COVID-19 vaccine may not have been possible. In 2023, Karikó and colleague Drew Weissman were awarded the 2023 Nobel Prize in Physiology or Medicine for their work on mRNA vaccines. Reflecting on her role in the development of COVID-19 vaccines, Karikó says, "[In 2020] I received my first dose together with Drew Weissman at the University of Pennsylvania. It was an incredible feeling to receive it, knowing well the composition and history of the vaccine. However, more overwhelming was hearing the feelings of relief and hope from others." Karikó also stresses the importance of never giving up. She says, "Like many scientists, I have faced a lot of challenges during my career, especially in terms of finding lab positions and obtaining grant funding. I kept going because I love being a researcher—the joy that you are the first person to learn something and that you finally see the picture that the puzzle pieces make up."

Quoted in Adam Gristwood, "Getting the Message Right: An Interview with mRNA Vaccine Pioneer Katalin Karikó," *EMBO Reports*, vol. 24, no. 11, November 2023. www.embopress.org.

Cutter Incident is one well-known example. In 1955, soon after the polio vaccine was approved, it was discovered that thousands of batches of vaccine that had been produced by Cutter Laboratories—one of five companies making the polio vaccine—unintentionally contained live polio virus, even though the batches had been tested for safety. It was estimated that about 220,000 people received theses vaccines before the contamination was discovered. The contaminated vaccines made many people sick. They caused muscle weakness in tens of thousands, paralyzed more than 160, and killed 10.

Laurie Maffly-Kipp says that three of her cousins received the contaminated vaccine. Although her cousins only experienced a mild case of sickness, her twenty-nine-year-old aunt caught it from them. Maffly-Kipp recalls, "She spent the following six months in an iron lung and nearly died. Her doctors told her that she might make it to age 30 but had little chance of surviving long with the damage to her lung capacity and swallowing muscles." Nonetheless, Maffly-Kipp explains that her aunt did live to age seventy; however, she lived with significant health problems throughout her life. Despite all of this, her aunt still believed in vaccination. "Millions of children lived long and healthy lives because of the polio vaccine,"[26] Maffly-Kipp says. The CDC notes that the Cutter Incident did result in improved safety procedures. It says, "The Cutter Incident was a defining moment in the history of vaccine manufacturing and government oversight of vaccines, and led to the creation of a better system of regulating vaccines."[27]

The RotaShield vaccine is another example of a vaccine that was approved for use but was later withdrawn because it was found to be harmful in a significant number of people. This vaccine was approved in 1998 for preventing rotavirus gastroenteritis, an infection that can cause severe vomiting and diarrhea. Its approval came after years of testing. However, soon after widespread infant vaccination began, reports indicated that some infants were experiencing intussusception, a type of bowel obstruction in which the intestine folds in on itself. This condition can cause serious health problems, including bleeding, infection, and death of intestinal tissue. An investigation revealed that the vaccine was linked to an increased risk of this condition in some infants. According to the CDC, after the first dose, the risk of infants developing intussusception was twenty to thirty times above the normal rate. Government recommendation for the vaccine was withdrawn, and the manufacturer took RotaShield off the market. The CDC reports that the number of infants vaccinated with RotaShield before it was withdrawn from the market is unknown. It only states that approximately seven thousand received it in testing before it was licensed, and "many more"[28] got it in the nine months before it was withdrawn.

The COVID-19 Vaccine

The development of the COVID-19 vaccine did not follow the usual timeline. Instead, this vaccine was developed much more quickly. Researchers were able to rapidly develop a COVID-19 vaccine because a lot of research had already been conducted on similar viruses. The university-affiliated health system UCLA Health explains,

> It's true that the trio of COVID-19 vaccines now in use in the U.S. became available at record speed. This is due, in no small part, to previous research that went into developing similar . . . vaccines. This includes vaccine development for MERS (Middle East respiratory syndrome) and SARS (severe acute respiratory syndrome), each of which are caused by a coronavirus. So when the call went out for a vaccine targeting the coronavirus that causes COVID-19, researchers weren't starting from scratch. They were building on decades of existing research and development.[29]

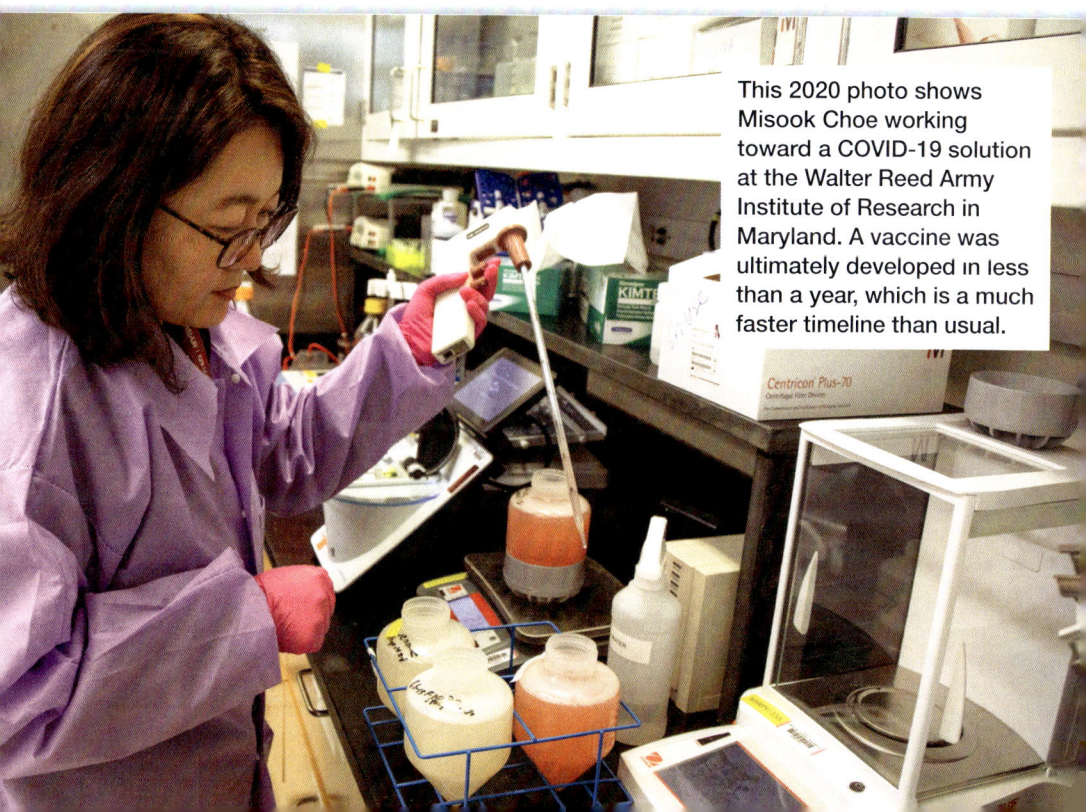

This 2020 photo shows Misook Choe working toward a COVID-19 solution at the Walter Reed Army Institute of Research in Maryland. A vaccine was ultimately developed in less than a year, which is a much faster timeline than usual.

Can Vaccine Manufacturers Be Trusted?

Pharmaceutical companies develop vaccines, test them, and then manufacture and sell them for a profit. Since these companies often make a lot of money from their vaccines, it is common for people to wonder whether they can trust the safety studies that have been conducted. Critics charge that pharmaceutical companies are focused on making money above all else and argue that it is a conflict of interest for these companies to be the ones conducting the safety studies concerning their products. Others contend that while pharmaceutical companies do conduct the studies, there are many other procedures to ensure that safety is not compromised. The Vaccine Education Center at Children's Hospital of Philadelphia says,

> In fact, many people, not just those who manufacture vaccines, study vaccine safety. The Food and Drug Administration (FDA) reviews all data associated with studies completed by vaccine manufacturers as well as visiting manufacturing sites and continuing to monitor the vaccine as long as it is being made. Additionally, the CDC has systems in place to monitor vaccine safety, of which vaccine manufacturers are not a part.

Vaccine Education Center, "Vaccine Science: Common Questions About Vaccine Liability," Children's Hospital of Philadelphia. www.chop.edu.

Vaccine development was also sped by an emergency use authorization from the FDA. This is an order that can be used to help accelerate the availability of certain medical products, such as vaccines, during a public health emergency. It can only be used when there are no better alternatives and when the potential benefits of the vaccine or other product outweigh the risks. Under an emergency use authorization, the review, approval, and manufacture of vaccines can be fast-tracked, as was the case with the COVID-19 vaccines. The FDA stresses that under this authorization, researchers and manufacturers still must follow strict testing and safety protocols. It maintains, "Efforts to speed vaccine development to address the ongoing COVID-19 pandemic have not sacrificed scientific standards, integrity of the vaccine review process, or safety."[30] For instance, the FDA maintains that the vaccine was still tested on tens of thousands of people before being approved and that safety monitoring is ongoing.

Finally, the US government helped accelerate the development of the vaccine by providing funding for that development. Stéphane Bancel is the chief executive officer of Moderna, which produced one of the first COVID-19 vaccines approved in the United States. He says, "We got a lot of help. . . . I really want to again, thank the US government. . . . We got funding, we got a lot of funding. . . . Moderna has got more than $1 billion, so we could take a lot [of] business risk[s] because that's the only way we could save time."[31] For instance, Bancel explains that in the regular process of vaccine development, a company does phase one testing and only starts investing resources in preparing for phase two after phase one is successful. However, with government funding for developing the COVID-19 vaccine, he says that Moderna was able to prepare for phase two while phase one was still in progress, which helped the company save a lot of time.

> "Efforts to speed vaccine development to address the ongoing COVID-19 pandemic have not sacrificed scientific standards, integrity of the vaccine review process, or safety."[30]
>
> —US Food and Drug Administration

New Vaccine Technology

The first two COVID-19 vaccines approved in the United States were mRNA vaccines, the first of this type to be approved for human use. All vaccines work by helping the body learn to recognize a particular virus so that it will be prepared to fight against that virus if necessary in the future. Traditional vaccines do this by putting dead or weakened virus inside the body. In contrast, mRNA vaccines do not contain actual virus. Instead, they work by giving a person's cells instructions on how to recognize and fight a particular virus. The body makes its own mRNA so that it can direct its cells to take different actions, including fighting disease.

Just like the mRNA humans produce naturally, the mRNA from the vaccines breaks down in the body in a few days.

Because the fight against COVID-19 was the first time that mRNA vaccines had been approved for human use, some people worry that there might be side effects that researchers have not yet had time to discover, especially since the COVID-19 vaccines were approved so quickly. In a research study that questioned people about their attitudes regarding the COVID-19 vaccine, one participant commented, "There was mass testing but it was over a shorter period of time than other vaccines had been. So, I think there could be so many side-effects in the long term that we don't know about. And we don't have time to find out about them."[32]

Researchers respond that while the COVID-19 vaccines are the first approved mRNA vaccines, the technology itself is not new. According to Pfizer, this technology was discovered during the 1960s and has been the subject of a lot of research since then. It says, "Scientists have been studying mRNA for decades."[33] Immunologist Sarah Fortune of the Harvard T.H. Chan School of

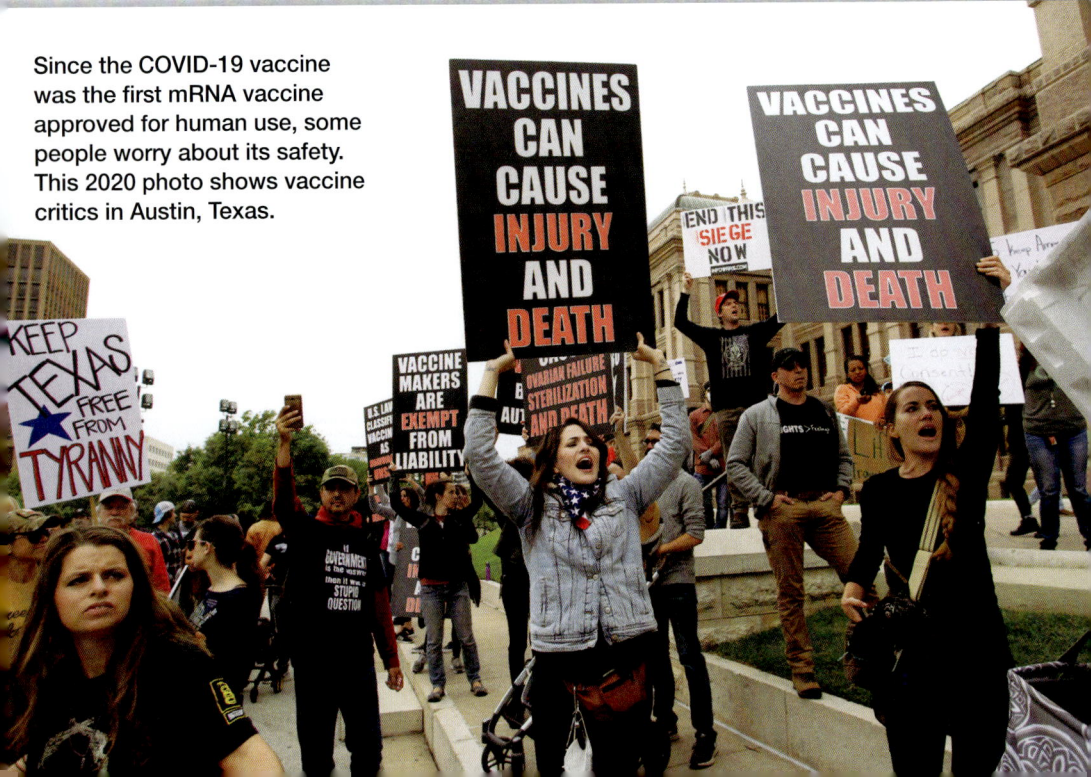

Since the COVID-19 vaccine was the first mRNA vaccine approved for human use, some people worry about its safety. This 2020 photo shows vaccine critics in Austin, Texas.

Public Health agrees. She says that, in fact, researchers have already used mRNA technology for other vaccines, but these are still in various stages of development. She adds, "It's not technically true that this is the first time that one of these vaccines has been produced. It's just it's the first time that one of these vaccines has made it through the full regulatory cycle and gone into people in large scale. So actually, the mRNA platforms have been used for both different infectious disease vaccines and cancer vaccines."[34]

As history reveals, there are no guarantees when it comes to vaccine safety. However, oversight has come a long way since the experimentation of Edward Jenner. In the United States and most other countries, there are strict regulations in place that are designed to ensure the highest level of safety possible. These regulations are based on years of research and experience. Overall, the HHS says, "Vaccines are some of the most studied medical interventions in the world."[35] While there have been some failures in the regulation process, there are also continued efforts to learn from and prevent similar failures in the future.

> "Vaccines are some of the most studied medical interventions in the world."[35]
>
> —US Department of Health and Human Services

CHAPTER FOUR

Vaccine Mandates

After the COVID-19 vaccine was approved in 2020, both governments and private companies in the United States enacted vaccine mandates. For instance, in September 2021, the federal government began to require vaccination for its employees. Many states also mandated vaccinations for certain groups of people, such as health care workers and nursing home employees. In addition, a significant number of private businesses required their employees to get vaccinated, and some—such as restaurants—refused to serve people without proof of vaccination. These mandates were very controversial. While some people were strongly in favor of them, others were adamant that mandates violated their personal freedom.

Danielle Thornton was one of thousands of people who lost their jobs after refusing to get vaccinated. Like many of the other people who objected to a vaccine mandate, she insisted, "I should have the right to choose." She says that she gave up her job because she and her husband agreed that "our freedom was more important than a pay cheque."[36] A Gallup poll conducted at the end of 2021 shows that although most Americans agreed with mandatory vaccination, a significant number did not. Of those polled, 55 percent were in favor of vaccination requirements at work, 35 percent were opposed, and 11 percent did not have an opinion. Vaccine mandates did not begin with the COVID-19 pandemic; instead, they have been around for more than a hundred years. And they have always been controversial.

Early Mandates

The earliest vaccine mandates were for the smallpox vaccine, which was the first vaccine to be developed. Public officials began requiring this vaccine in order to eradicate smallpox, which was causing devastating outbreaks around the world. During the Revolutionary War, George Washington's Continental Army battled both the British Army and smallpox. By 1777, his forces were so wrecked by smallpox that he required all soldiers to be vaccinated. According to a National Park Service article, Washington called smallpox "more destructive than the sword."[37] In 1809, Massachusetts issued the first state vaccine mandate, requiring that adults over age twenty-one be vaccinated against smallpox. Many other states followed.

Even in the early days of vaccine mandates, there were vocal opponents to these policies. The Anti-Vaccination Society of America was founded in 1879 and was followed by several other organizations against mandatory vaccination. These organizations fought to have vaccine mandates repealed, in some cases successfully. Many of the early arguments against vaccine mandates were based on fears that vaccination was not safe and on the belief that the government did not have the right to make decisions about people's health. Some people argued that outbreaks were only a problem in poor communities that struggled with overcrowding and unsanitary conditions, and these objectors believed that they could avoid getting smallpox simply by keeping themselves clean and healthy. Journalist Tara Haelle sums up common anti-vaccine beliefs at that time, stating, "Anti-vaccination groups argued that compulsory vaccination violated personal liberty, writing that the acts 'trample upon the right of parents to protect their children from disease' and 'invaded liberty by rendering good health a crime.'"[38]

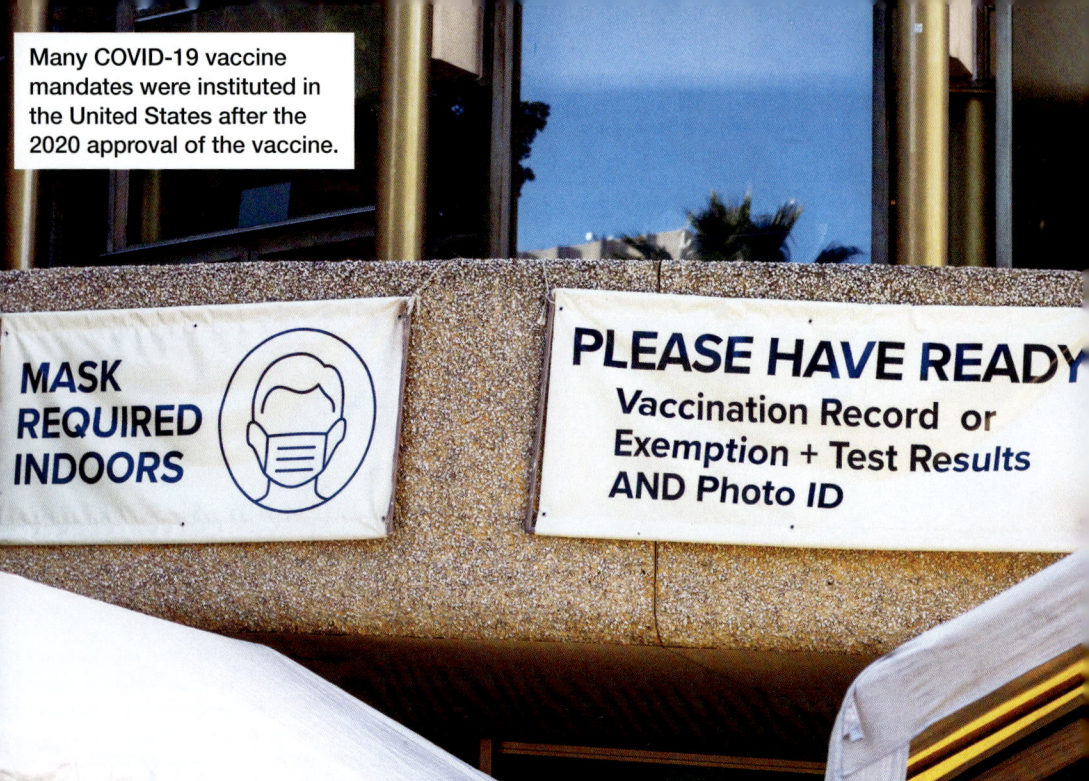

Many COVID-19 vaccine mandates were instituted in the United States after the 2020 approval of the vaccine.

In 1905, the debate over vaccine mandates went all the way to the US Supreme Court, which ruled that the government does have the authority to mandate vaccination. In this case, a Massachusetts man did not want to receive a government-mandated smallpox vaccine, arguing that forcing him to do so was a violation of his personal freedom. The court disagreed. In its 1905 *Jacobson v. Massachusetts* ruling, it stressed that while personal freedom is important, in some cases—such as with the smallpox vaccine—the good of the public is more important. It stated,

> The liberty secured by the Constitution of the United States to every person within its jurisdiction does not import an absolute right in each person to be, at all times and in all circumstances, wholly freed from restraint. There are manifold restraints to which every person is necessarily subject for the common good. On any other basis organized society could not exist with safety to its members.[39]

Childhood Vaccines

Many early vaccine mandates applied specifically to children. In 1855, Massachusetts became the first US state to require that children receive a smallpox vaccine before they could attend school. There was a yearly fine for parents who did not vaccinate their children. Many states followed Massachusetts's example. Over time, additional vaccines were added to the list of required childhood vaccines, and more states passed mandates. By 1963, twenty states had vaccine requirements for schoolchildren. By the 1998 to 1999 school year, all states except four (Louisiana, Michigan, South Carolina, and West Virginia) had vaccine mandates for children in kindergarten through twelfth grade. At present, all fifty states plus the District of Columbia require that children and teens be vaccinated against diphtheria, tetanus, pertussis, polio, measles, rubella, and chicken pox. All but Iowa mandate vaccination for mumps. While individual states make their own rules, the CDC makes recommendations about the vaccines that children should receive. In total, it now recommends sixteen different vaccinations; however, not all of these are mandated by state governments.

Over time, the number of vaccines on the CDC's list has increased substantially. In the late 1940s, only four vaccines were recommended: smallpox, diphtheria, tetanus, and pertussis. In the 1950s, the polio vaccine was added, and in the 1960s, measles, mumps, and rubella were included, with the total number of recommended vaccinations reaching eight. Since then, new vaccines continue to be added to the list, which has doubled in size since the 1960s. Some people worry about the effects of children receiving so many vaccines. However, the Vaccine Education Center at Children's Hospital of Philadelphia explains that although the number of vaccines has increased, due to technological innovation, vaccines have become much more advanced, and children are actually being exposed to less immunological components. The center says,

> In the late 1980s and early 1990s, children received vaccines that protected against eight diseases: measles, mumps, rubella, diphtheria, tetanus, pertussis, Haemophilus influenzae type b and polio. The total number of bacterial and viral proteins contained in these vaccines was a little more than 3,000. Today, children receive vaccines that protect against 14 diseases, but the total number of immunological components in these vaccines is only about 150. This dramatic reduction is the result of scientific advances in protein chemistry and protein purification that have allowed for purer, safer vaccines.[40]

Current Vaccine Mandates

At present, most vaccine mandates in the United States are for children. Vaccine mandates for adults have become less common than in the early days of the smallpox vaccine. Some states, though, do mandate specific vaccines for certain adults. For example, in Rhode Island, both health care workers and child care workers must be immunized against several diseases, including chicken pox, measles, mumps, rubella, and the flu. In New York, college students are required to show proof of MMR vaccination. Many states also passed COVID-19 vaccine mandates during the pandemic, but some of those have been removed.

The United States is not the only country with vaccine mandates. Many other countries have vaccine mandates for children, including the Czech Republic, France, Hungary, Italy, and Poland. However, there are also many

> "Scientific advances in protein chemistry and protein purification . . . have allowed for purer, safer vaccines."[40]
>
> —Vaccine Education Center at Children's Hospital of Philadelphia

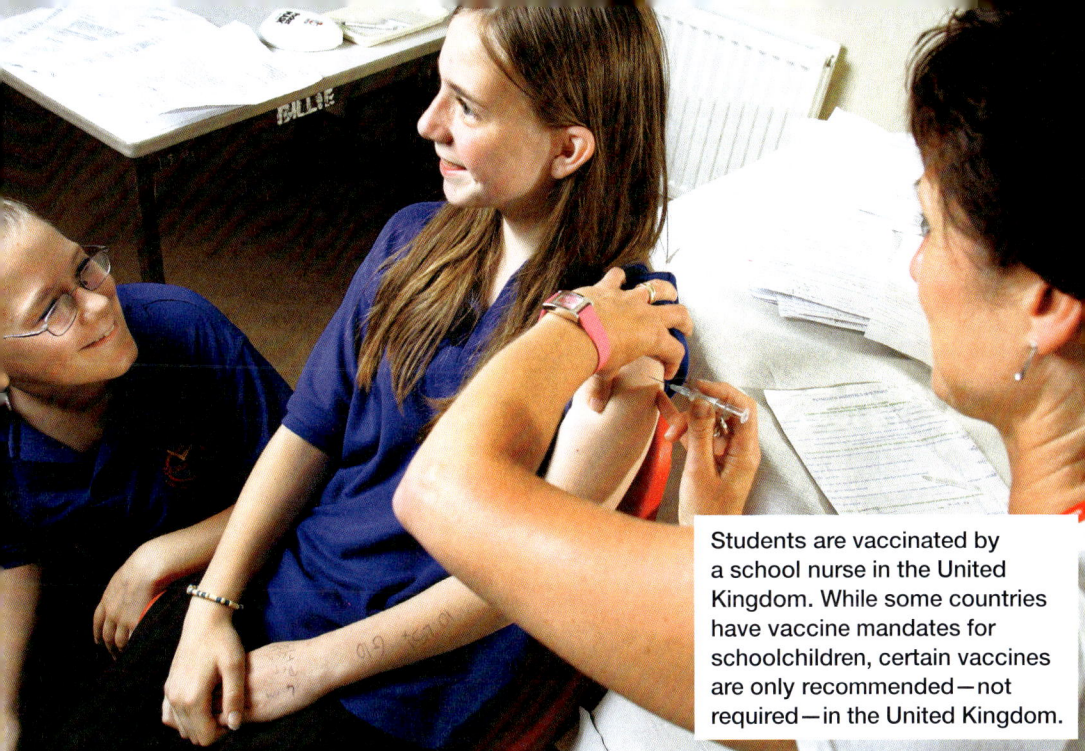

Students are vaccinated by a school nurse in the United Kingdom. While some countries have vaccine mandates for schoolchildren, certain vaccines are only recommended—not required—in the United Kingdom.

countries—such as Netherlands, New Zealand, Switzerland, and the United Kingdom—in which certain vaccines are recommended for children but are not required. In Canada, childhood vaccines are not mandatory, yet they are required in some provinces. As with the United States, many countries passed COVID-19 vaccination mandates during the pandemic, but some have begun to remove those requirements post pandemic.

Vaccine Exemptions

When it comes to vaccine mandates, most countries allow exceptions for certain groups of people. These vaccine exemptions occur when people opt out of vaccination for themselves or their children due to medical, religious, or other reasons. In the United States, specific types of allowed exemptions vary by state, and in most cases, they are used to opt out of childhood vaccines. Medical exemptions are very common, especially when a particular vaccine might be unsafe for a child. For instance, that child

Mandates May Increase Opposition to Vaccination

Some people are opposed to vaccine mandates not because they do not believe in vaccination but rather because they believe that trying to force people to get vaccinated can decrease vaccination rates. Researchers explain the psychological theory behind this: "Individuals appreciate behavioral freedom. When freedom is restricted . . . individuals will experience reactance, a composite of anger and negative cognitions motivating them to regain the freedom lost." In many cases, this means refusing to get vaccinated. These researchers studied two groups of people—in Germany and the United States—to gain a better understanding of COVID-19 vaccine mandates. They found that mandates were more likely to increase anti-vaccine activism and reduce the likelihood that people would get vaccinated, both for COVID-19 and for illnesses in the future.

Philipp Sprengholz, Cornelia Betsch, and Robert Böhm, "Reactance Revisited: Consequences of Mandatory and Scarce Vaccination in the Case of COVID-19," *Applied Psychology: Health and Well-Being*, vol. 13, no. 4, November 2021. https://pmc.ncbi.nlm.nih.gov.

might have had a severe reaction to a vaccine in the past, might be allergic to an ingredient in the vaccine, or might have a weakened immune system.

With a religious or personal exemption, parents can opt out of having their child vaccinated because it conflicts with their beliefs. Religious and personal objections to vaccination are relatively common and vary widely. One example of a personal objection to a vaccine is in relation to the human papillomavirus (HPV) vaccine, which was first approved in the United States in 2006. This vaccine protects against HPV, which can cause cancer. After it was approved, some states tried to mandate vaccinations of young people, but a significant number of parents objected. Though many cited safety concerns, some objections were based on personal belief. This virus is spread through sexual activity, and they felt that vaccinating their children would discourage them from limiting their sexual behavior or remaining abstinent.

Opinions About Exemptions

In 2024, the CDC surveyed more than two thousand parents about mandatory vaccines for their children and found that 3.8 percent of respondents had obtained an exemption in the past. Among these respondents, the most common reasons for exemption were philosophical or personal beliefs (37.5 percent), medical reasons (27.2 percent), and trouble meeting school requirement deadlines (22.6 percent). In recent years, there has been an increase in the number of people applying for exemptions for their children and an overall decrease in the percentage of school-age children who are vaccinated. As a result, there have been concerns that herd immunity is being compromised, and some states have tried to get rid of personal belief exemptions. California successfully did so in 2016. Maine removed both personal and religious exemptions in 2019.

Medical exemptions are generally not controversial, but there are strong opinions about other types of exemptions. On one side of the debate are people who believe that everyone should have the ability to exempt themselves or their children from vaccination if it goes against their beliefs. New Jersey mother Jessica Milner is a strong advocate of allowing people to exempt their children from vaccines due to religious and personal beliefs. "Whenever there is a risk of any kind, there needs to be a choice in the matter," she insists. "Vaccines are a medical procedure, and there is a risk in any medical procedure, so there needs to be true and informed consent, and choice."[41] Maine mother Sarah Staffiere is more skeptical. Her young son is on medication that inactivates his immune system, which means that it is risky for him to be around unvaccinated children. "Any hard-hitting illness that he receives could lead him to develop complications that other kids wouldn't," says

> "Whenever there is a risk of any kind, there needs to be a choice in the matter."[41]
>
> —Jessica Milner, New Jersey mother

Staffiere. "For him, just getting the flu can be quite scary. My hope is that he would be surrounded by as many vaccinated kids as possible, to keep him in as healthy an environment as possible."[42]

Mandates and Personal Freedom

Many arguments related to vaccine mandates are centered on the idea of personal freedom and whether people should have the freedom to decline vaccination if they disagree with it or if they should be forced to vaccinate to protect public health. Vaccine mandates are implemented to protect the health of the community. By forcing most community members to become vaccinated, herd immunity is achieved, which makes it much more difficult for infectious diseases to exist in that community. Supporters of vaccine mandates insist that although personal freedom is a defining part of being an American, in this case, public health trumps individual freedom. Epidemiologist Elizabeth Miller explains, "While individual freedom of choice is an important principle, those who refuse vaccination not only pose a risk to themselves but also to others."[43] The American Civil Liberties Union agrees. Citing COVID-19 vaccine mandates, it maintains that whereas people do have the right to make choices about their bodies, they do not have the right to harm other people by refusing to get vaccinated. It says, "In fact, far from compromising civil liberties, vaccine mandates actually *further* civil liberties. They protect the most vulnerable among us."[44]

However, critics contend that forcing people to get vaccinated infringes on their individual freedom. In 2021, Guam's governor signed an executive order mandating COVID-19 vaccinations for executive branch government workers, which was met with protest. Protester Paul Burton insisted, "This is a matter of freedom and human dignity. Even if the vaccine is safe and completely necessary, that does not give her the right to deprive individuals of their personal freedom. . . . No government leader has the right or constitutional authority to mandate medical procedures to private citizens."⁴⁵

Growing Resistance to Mandates

In recent years, there has been growing opposition to vaccine mandates. Some opponents are well-known celebrities or politicians, and their voices have helped the anti-vaccine movement grow. For instance, in 2024 politician Robert F. Kennedy Jr. opposed mandatory vaccination, saying, "People ought to have choice."⁴⁶ As a result of growing resistance to vaccine mandates, in some places, the number of children being vaccinated has declined significantly. The CDC reports that vaccination for measles, mumps, rubella, diphtheria, tetanus, pertussis, polio, and chicken pox has declined from 95 percent—which is what researchers say is needed for herd immunity—to approximately 93 percent.

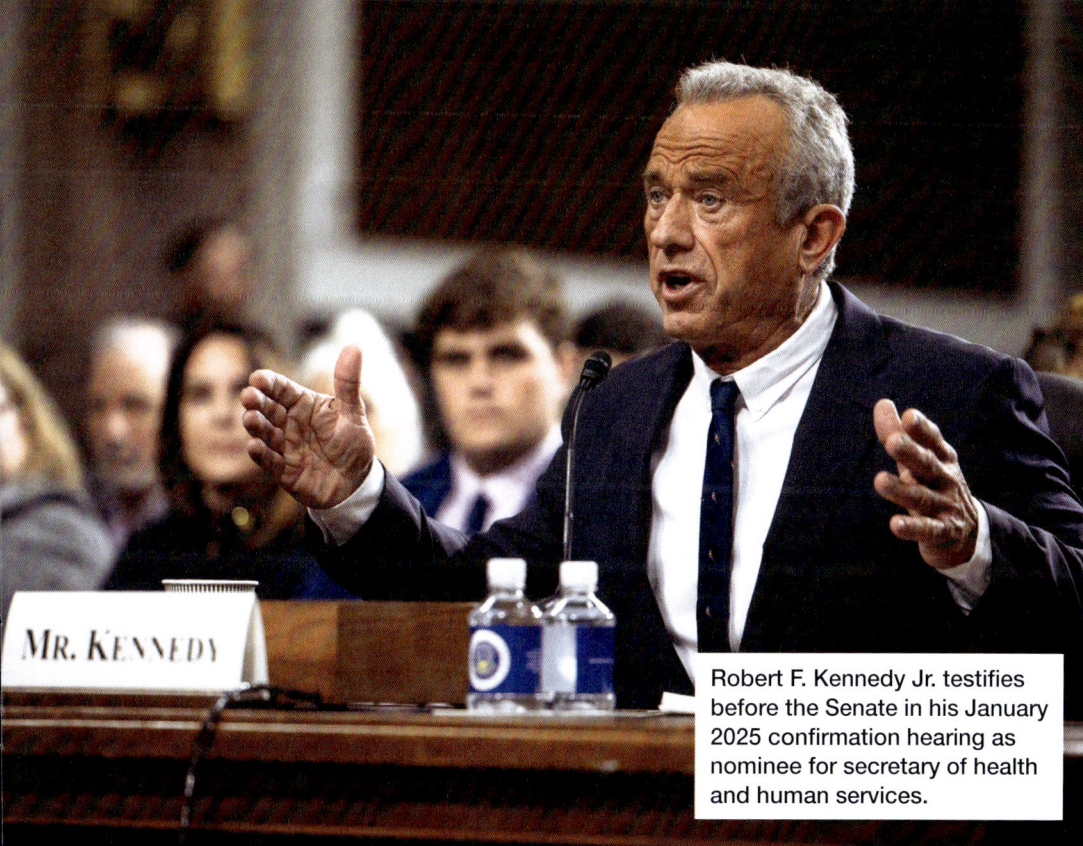

Robert F. Kennedy Jr. testifies before the Senate in his January 2025 confirmation hearing as nominee for secretary of health and human services.

Experts warn that as more people refuse to vaccinate themselves or their children, illnesses that have not threatened society in a long time may return.

This seems to be happening with measles. Measles causes a fever, cough, and itchy rash, but it can also result in serious complications like pneumonia or swelling of the brain and can even lead to death. It is very contagious. In both the United States and Europe, cases of measles have increased in the past few years. The CDC reported that there were more than 10.3 million cases of measles worldwide in 2023. This marked an increase of 20 percent from 2022. It says, "Inadequate immunization coverage globally is driving the surge in cases."[47] In the past, measles was thought to have been almost eliminated from the United States, but there have been several recent outbreaks of this disease. Jessica Coletti's three-year-old son, Vincent, caught this illness in 2024. She worried that her unvaccinated infant daughter might also get sick, and she and her husband had to stay home until they could prove that they were not sick. Coletti says, "The night-

Distrust of Health Care

Some people are opposed to vaccine mandates because they generally distrust the health care system. Researchers have found that in the United States, distrust is more common among people of color, and they explain that this is likely because this community has historically been mistreated and discriminated against by that system. The Commonwealth Fund, an organization that works to improve the US health care system, explains that "the medical establishment has a long history of mistreating Black Americans—from gruesome experiments on enslaved people to the forced sterilizations of Black women and the infamous Tuskegee syphilis study that withheld treatment from hundreds of Black men for decades to let doctors track the course of the disease." At the beginning of the COVID-19 pandemic, researchers found that opposition to vaccination was high among Black communities.

Martha Hostetter and Sarah Klein, "Understanding and Ameliorating Medical Mistrust Among Black Americans," Commonwealth Fund, January 14, 2021. www.commonwealthfund.org.

mare wasn't just that my son was sick. That was horrible, but then it's your whole world. You can't go to work. You can't do this and that, and you can't even believe it."[48]

Mandates—and vaccines in general—continue to provoke widespread debate, with passionate arguments on both sides. Even people who are in favor of vaccination stress that it is not without risks. Epidemiologist Elizabeth Miller maintains, "Concern about vaccine safety is . . . perfectly legitimate."[49] However, there are also many risks that come with not vaccinating. Choosing whether to undergo vaccination is a process of comparing the risks with the benefits. Public health agencies around the world stress that in most cases, the benefits of vaccination outweigh the risks. All people, though, have the right to investigate this important topic for themselves.

> "Concern about vaccine safety is . . . perfectly legitimate."[49]
>
> —Elizabeth Miller, epidemiologist

SOURCE NOTES

Introduction: A Public Health Triumph
1. Quoted in Rachel Sanders and Anne Helen Peterson, "12 Teens on Being Stuck at Home Because of the Coronavirus," BuzzFeed News, March 19, 2020. www.buzzfeednews.com.

Chapter One: How Important Is Vaccination?
2. Quoted in Vaccine Education Center, "Parents PACK Personal Stories: Polio," Children's Hospital of Philadelphia. www.chop.edu.
3. Quoted in Vaccine Education Center, "Born Almost Deaf, Karen Did Not Let Rubella Define Her," Children's Hospital of Philadelphia. www.chop.edu.
4. Quoted in World Health Organization, "Global Immunization Efforts Have Saved at Least 154 Million Lives over the Past 50 Years," April 24, 2024. www.who.int.
5. Quoted in World Health Organization, "Global Immunization Efforts Have Saved at Least 154 Million Lives over the Past 50 Years."
6. National Foundation for Infectious Diseases, "10 Reasons to Get Vaccinated," 2024. www.nfid.org.
7. World Health Organization, "Vaccines and Immunization: Myths and Misconceptions," October 19, 2020. www.who.int.
8. Centers for Disease Control and Prevention, "Mumps Vaccination," January 17, 2025. www.cdc.gov.
9. World Health Organization, "Vaccines and Immunization."
10. US Department of Health and Human Services, "How Do We Know Vaccines Work?," December 19, 2024. www.hhs.gov.
11. Quoted in Dan Dean and Ronit Rose, "The Vaccine Controversy," Chicago Health, April 8, 2024. https://chicagohealthonline.com.

Chapter Two: Vaccine Side Effects
12. Quoted in Hannah Chinn, "The Rarest of COVID Vaccine Reactions: One Woman's Story of Guillain-Barre," WHYY, April 25, 2021. https://whyy.org.
13. Jonathan Jarry, "I Felt Sick After Getting a Vaccine. Why?," Office for Science and Society, McGill University, April 9, 2021. www.mcgill.ca.
14. World Health Organization, "Vaccines and Immunization."
15. Tina, "Stories: Vaccines Caused My Daughter's Seizures," Oregonians for Medical Freedom. www.oregoniansformedicalfreedom.com.

16. Health Resources and Services Administration, "Data & Statistics," January 1, 2025. www.hrsa.gov/sites/default/files/hrsa/advisory-committees/vaccines/vicp-stats-01-01-25.pdf.
17. Apoorva Mandavilli, "Thousands Believe Covid Vaccines Harmed Them. Is Anyone Listening?," *New York Times,* May 3, 2024. www.nytimes.com.
18. Quoted in Mandavilli, "Thousands Believe Covid Vaccines Harmed Them."
19. Quoted in World Health Organization, "'For Me, Long COVID Was Life Destroying': Eric, a Vicar from the UK, on How Rehabilitation Services Gave Him Hope," November 17, 2023. www.who.int.
20. US Food and Drug Administration, "Common Ingredients in FDA-Approved Vaccines," January 12, 2024. www.fda.gov.
21. American Academy of Allergy, Asthma & Immunology, "Vaccines: The Myths and the Facts," January 10, 2024. www.aaaai.org.
22. World Health Organization, "Vaccines and Immunization."

Chapter Three: Vaccine Safety

23. Quoted in Poppy Brown et al., "'It Seems Impossible That It's Been Made So Quickly': A Qualitative Investigation of Concerns About the Speed of COVID-19 Vaccine Development and How These May Be Overcome," *Human Vaccines & Immunotherapeutics*, vol. 18, no. 1, December 2022. https://pmc.ncbi.nlm.nih.gov.
24. Quoted in Brown et al., "'It Seems Impossible That It's Been Made So Quickly.'"
25. Richard Hollingham, "The Chilling Experiment Which Created the First Vaccine," British Broadcasting Corporation, September 29, 2020. www.bbc.com.
26. Laurie Maffly-Kipp, "The Infamous 'Cutter Vaccine' Changed My Family Forever—but We Still Support Vaccination," STAT, January 15, 2025. www.statnews.com.
27. Centers for Disease Control and Prevention, "Historical Vaccine Concerns," July 31, 2024. www.cdc.gov.
28. CDC Archive, "Rotavirus Vaccine (RotaShield) and Intussusception," April 22, 2011. https://archive.cdc.gov.
29. UCLA Health, "Vaccine Emergency-Use Authorization Speeds Up Availability," July 19, 2021. www.uclahealth.org.
30. US Food and Drug Administration, "Emergency Use Authorization for Vaccines Explained," November 20, 2020. www.fda.gov.
31. Quoted in Alexis Pedrick, "Interview with Stéphane Bancel," Science History Institute Museum & Library, June 7, 2021. www.sciencehistory.org.
32. Quoted in Brown et al., "'It Seems Impossible That It's Been Made So Quickly.'"
33. Pfizer, "Unleashing the Next Wave of Scientific Innovations to Fight Viruses and More." www.pfizer.com.

34. Quoted in Anna Fisher-Pinkert, "We're Better Off with mRNA Vaccines," Harvard T.H. Chan School of Public Health, February 24, 2021. https://hsph.harvard.edu.
35. US Department of Health and Human Services, "The Real Research Behind Vaccine Safety," Let's Get Real, December 19, 2024. www.hhs.gov.

Chapter Four: Vaccine Mandates

36. Quoted in Natalie Sherman, "Vaccine Mandates: 'I Lost My Job for Being Unvaccinated,'" British Broadcasting Corporation, January 23, 2022. www.bbc.com.
37. Quoted in Boston National Historical Park, "Smallpox, Inoculation, and the Revolutionary War," National Park Service. www.nps.gov.
38. Tara Haelle, "Vaccine Hesitancy Is Nothing New. Here's the Damage It's Done over Centuries," *Science News*, May 11, 2021. www.sciencenews.org.
39. US Supreme Court, "Jacobson v. Massachusetts, 197 U.S. 11 (1905)," Justia U.S. Supreme Court Center. https://supreme.justia.com.
40. Vaccine Education Center, "Too Many Vaccines? What You Should Know," Children's Hospital of Philadelphia, 2018. www.chop.edu.
41. Quoted in Roni Caryn Rabin, "Eager to Limit Exemptions to Vaccination, States Face Staunch Resistance," *New York Times,* June 14, 2019. www.nytimes.com.
42. Quoted in Rabin, "Eager to Limit Exemptions to Vaccination, States Face Staunch Resistance."
43. Elizabeth Miller, "Controversies and Challenges of Vaccination: An Interview with Elizabeth Miller," *BMC Medicine,* vol. 13, no. 267, October 16, 2015. https://bmcmedicine.biomedcentral.com.
44. David Cole and Daniel Mach, "Civil Liberties and Vaccine Mandates: Here's Our Take," American Civil Liberties Union, September 2, 2021. www.aclu.org.
45. Quoted in Mar-Vic Cagurangan, "Doctor Says Forced Vaccine Mandate 'Is a Slippery Slope to Totalitarianism,'" *Pacific Island Times* (Tumon, Guam)*,* August 24, 2021. www.pacificislandtimes.com.
46. Quoted in Vaughn Hillyard and Rebecca Shabad, "After Trump Win, RFK Jr. Says He Won't 'Take Away Anybody's Vaccines,'" NBC News, November 6, 2024. www.nbcnews.com.
47. Centers for Disease Control and Prevention, "Measles Cases Surge Worldwide, Infecting 10.3 Million People in 2023," November 14, 2024. www.cdc.gov.
48. Quoted in Jen Christensen, "Mother of Chicago Child with Measles: It Was 'One of the Scarier Moments of My Life,'" CNN, April 22, 2024. www.cnn.com.
49. Miller, "Controversies and Challenges of Vaccination."

ORGANIZATIONS AND WEBSITES

Centers for Disease Control and Prevention (CDC)
www.cdc.gov
As the national public health agency, the CDC is responsible for protecting the public health of Americans. Its website has many different vaccine-related resources, including fact sheets on individual vaccines, information about how vaccines work and how they are regulated, and statistics about use and safety.

Gavi, the Vaccine Alliance
www.gavi.org
Gavi is an international organization that works to increase the use of vaccines, including improving access to lower-income countries. Its website has news and information about vaccines, including success stories and details about emerging threats.

Immunize.org
www.immunize.org
Immunize.org is a nonprofit organization that works to advance knowledge about vaccination among the public and health care professionals. Its website contains a wide range of vaccine-related information. This includes guidance about recommended vaccines, including vaccines for travel; a vaccine history timeline; and information specific to individual vaccines.

US Food and Drug Administration (FDA)
www.fda.gov
The FDA is responsible for the regulation of vaccines in the United States. Its website has information about vaccine safety and side effects, including information about the COVID-19 vaccine. It also provides information about the other ingredients commonly found in vaccines and about the development and manufacturing process for vaccines.

Vaccine Education Center at Children's Hospital of Philadelphia
www.chop.edu/vaccine-education-center
This website, which has been approved as a vaccine resource by WHO, contains information on many vaccine-related topics. It has information about vaccine safety, the diseases that vaccines prevent, and vaccine science and history.

World Health Organization (WHO)
www.who.int
WHO is a United Nations agency dedicated to protecting and improving public health. Its website contains many different publications about how vaccines work, vaccine safety, and the impact of vaccination on public health.

FOR FURTHER RESEARCH

Books

John Allen, *Vaccine Wars: When Science and Politics Collide*. San Diego: ReferencePoint, 2022.

Maya J. Goldenberg, *Vaccine Hesitancy: Public Trust, Expertise, and the War on Science.* Pittsburgh: University of Pittsburgh Press, 2021.

Joe Miller, Özlem Türeci, and Uğur Şahin, *The Vaccine: Inside the Race to Conquer the COVID-19 Pandemic.* New York: St. Martin's, 2022.

Kimberley Tolley, *Vaccine Wars: The Two-Hundred-Year Fight for School Vaccinations*. Baltimore: Johns Hopkins University Press, 2023.

Internet Sources

American Academy of Allergy, Asthma & Immunology, "Vaccines: The Myths and the Facts," January 10, 2024. www.aaaai.org.

Centers for Disease Control and Prevention, "How Vaccines Are Developed and Approved for Use," August 10, 2024. www.cdc.gov.

Immunize.org, "Vaccine History Timeline," July 5, 2024. www.immunize.org.

Vaccine Education Center, "Vaccines and Diseases," Children's Hospital of Philadelphia, July 18, 2022. www.chop.edu.

World Health Organization, "Vaccines and Immunization: What Is Vaccination?," April 23, 2024. www.who.int.

INDEX

Note: Boldface page numbers indicate illustrations.

adverse side effects
  allergic reactions, 21–22
  GBS, 20
  prevalence of, 23
  programs tracking, 23–24
  to COVID-19 vaccine, 24–27
allergic reactions, 21
American Academy of Allergy, Asthma & Immunology, 28
American Civil Liberties Union, 50
Anti-Vaccination Society of America, 43
autism, MMR vaccine and, 28–30

Black Americans, distrust of health care system among, 52
Bossward, Eric, 26
British Broadcasting Corporation, 33
Burton, Paul, 50–51

Center for Biologics Evaluation and Research, 33
Centers for Disease Control and Prevention (CDC), 7, 57
  on diphtheria, 13
  on prevalence of GBS, 21
  on RotaShield vaccine, 36
  on steps in vaccine development, 33
  on surge in measles cases, 52
  on whooping cough vaccines, 16, 17
chicken pox, 17, 45, 46, 51

Choe, Misook, **37**
Cleveland Clinic, 15
Coletti, Jessica, 52–53
Commonwealth Fund, 52
Countermeasures Injury Compensation Program, 24–25
COVID-19 infection
  GBS following, 27
COVID-19 pandemic, 4–5
COVID-19 vaccine
  approval of, 31
  FDA's emergency use authorization for, 38–39
  lives saved by, 4
  myocarditis and, 29
  need for, after having had COVID-19, 15
  prior research speeding development of, 37
  side effects associated with, 24–27
  side effects of, 20
cowpox, 32
Cruz-Esteves, Rebeca, 20
Cutter Incident/Cutter Laboratories, 34–36

Department of Health and Human Services, US (HHS), 15–16, 17, 41
diphtheria, 13, 46
  See also DTaP
diseases, eradicated, 14–15
DTaP (diphtheria/tetanus/pertussis) vaccine, 16–17

encephalitis, 21–22

Food and Drug Administration, US (FDA), 24, 33, 57
   vaccine safety monitored by, 34
formaldehyde, 27–28
Fortune, Sarah, 40–41

Gallup poll, 42
Gavi, the Vaccine Alliance, 57
GBS. *See* Guillain-Barré syndrome
Ghebreyesus, Tedros Adhanom, 10–11
Guillain-Barré syndrome (GBS), 20
   after COVID-19 infection, 27

Haelle, Tara, 43
Haemophilus influenzae, 46
Hazra, Aniruddha, 18
health care system, distrust of, 52
Health Resources and Services Administration (HRSA), 24
hepatitis B, 9
herd immunity
   diseases not possible to achieve, 13
   vaccination mandates and, 49
   vaccination rates needed to achieve, 50
human papillomavirus (HPV) vaccine, 48

immune system, 5
immunity, 5
   natural, 14
   See also herd immunity
influenza vaccine, 21, 46
   herd immunity not achievable for, 13
iron lung, **10**, 36
Iwasaki, Akiko, 29

Jacobson v. Massachusetts (1905), 44
Jarry, Jonathan, 21
Jenner, Edward, 6–7, 31–32, **32**, 41
Johnson, Noelle, 4

Karikó, Katalin, 35
Kennedy, Robert F., Jr., 51, **51**

Lancet (journal), 4, 29
long COVID, 25
   prevalence of, 26

Maffly-Kipp, Laurie, 35–36
mandates, vaccination
   COVID-19 vaccine, 47
   exceptions to, 47–48
   for childhood vaccines, 45–46
   growing resistance to, 51–53
   medical exceptions to, 49
   personal freedom and, 50–51
   public opinion on, 49–50
   religious/personal exceptions to, 47–48
Mandavilli, Apoorva, 24
measles, 46
   mandates for vaccination against, 45
   recent surge in, 52
   vaccination rate needed for herd immunity against, 13
   See also MMR
meningococcal disease, 9
messenger ribonucleic acid (mRNA), 5–6
   See also mRNA vaccines
Miller, Elizabeth, 50, 53
Milner, Jessica, 49
MMR (measles/mumps/rubella) vaccine, 14, 17, 46

autism and, 28–29
mRNA vaccines, 5–6, 29, 35, 41
   COVID-19 vaccine as first,
     39–40
mumps, 46
   mandates for vaccination
     against, 45
   See also MMR
myocarditis, 29

National Foundation for Infectious
   Diseases (NFID), 11
National Park Service, 43

opinion polls. *See* surveys

pertussis (whooping cough), 16,
   46, 51
   See also DTaP
Pfizer, 29, 40
polio/polio vaccine, 8, 9
   mandates for, 45
   safety failure with, 34–36
polls. *See* surveys
public opinion
   on vaccination, 18–19
   on vaccine mandates, 49–50
   See also surveys

research studies
   on potential side effects of
     vaccines, 7
RotaShield vaccine, 36
rotavirus gastroenteritis, 36
rubella, 9
   See also MMR
Russell, Catherine, 11

Sadler, Karen, 9–10

safety failures, 34–36
Salk, Jonas, 9
smallpox/smallpox vaccine, 6–7,
   12, 32–33
   mandate for, 43–44, 46
Staffiere, Sarah, 49–50
surveys
   on attitudes toward vaccination,
     18
   on vaccine mandates, 42

Tdap (tetanus/diphtheria/
   pertussis) vaccine, 16–17
tetanus, 45, 46, 51
   See also DTaP
thimerosal, 27, 28
Thornton, Danielle, 42
Tuskegee syphilis study, 52

UCLA Health, 37
United Nations Children's Fund
   (UNICEF), 18

vaccination
   access to, 18
   as causing illness, 17
   community benefits of, 11–12
   first successful, 31–33
   people not eligible for, 11–12
   public opinion on, 18–19
   reasons people get sick after
     having, 15–17
   See also mandates
Vaccine Adverse Event Reporting
   System (VAERS), 23, 34
Vaccine Education Center
   (Children's Hospital of
   Philadelphia), 38, 45, 46, 57

Vaccine Injury Compensation Program, 23–24
vaccines
  assessing risks *vs.* benefits of, 30
  controversy over, 7
  ingredients, safety of, 27–28
  mechanism of, 5–7
  negative side effects of, 20–24
  process of developing, 33–34
  reduction in immunological components in, 46
  whooping cough, 16–17

Wakefield, Andrew, 28–29
Washington, George, 43
Weissman, Drew, 35
whooping cough (pertussis), 16, 46, 51
  See also DTaP
Woodcock, Janet, 24
World Health Organization (WHO), 10, 11, 58
  on global spread of disease, 15
  on prevalence of serious adverse reactions, 22
  on risks *vs.* benefits of vaccines, 30

PICTURE CREDITS

Cover: Alexander Raths/Shutterstock

6: Basilico Studio Stock/Shutterstock
10: Gado Images/Alamy Stock Photo
12: David Cole/Alamy Stock Photo
16: DimaBerlin/Shutterstock
22: Kmpzzz/Shutterstock
26: dpa picture alliance/Alamy Stock Photo
28: thodonal88/Shutterstock
32: Pictuers Now/Alamy Stock Photo
37: AC NewsPhoto/Alamy Stock Photo
40: Vic Hinterlang/Shutterstock
44: Michael Vi/Alamy Stock Photo
47: Marc Hill/Alamy Stock Photo
51: Associated Press

ABOUT THE AUTHOR

Andrea C. Nakaya, a native of New Zealand, holds a bachelor of arts in English and a master of arts in communications from San Diego State University. She has written and edited numerous articles and more than fifty books on current issues. She currently lives in Eagle, Idaho.